$\mathcal{A}$ DAYBOOK
for Critical Care Nurses

Eileen Gallen Bademan, BSN, RN

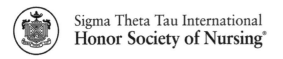

Sigma Theta Tau International
Honor Society of Nursing®

In collaboration with

AMERICAN
ASSOCIATION
of CRITICAL-CARE
NURSES

Sigma Theta Tau International
550 West North Street
Indianapolis, IN 46202

To order additional books, buy in bulk, or order for corporate use, contact Nursing Knowledge International at 888.NKI.4YOU (888.654.4968/US and Canada) or +1.317.634.8171 (outside US and Canada).

To request a review copy for course adoption, e-mail solutions@nursingknowledge.org or call 888.NKI.4YOU (888.654.4968/US and Canada) or +1.317.917.4983 (outside US and Canada).

To request author information, or for speaker or other media requests, contact Rachael McLaughlin of the Honor Society of Nursing, Sigma Theta Tau International at 888.634.7575 (US and Canada) or +1.317.634.8171 (outside US and Canada).

ISBN-13: 978-1-930538-89-4

Library of Congress Cataloging-in-Publication Data

Bademan, Eileen Gallen, 1963-
    A daybook for critical care nurses / Eileen Gallen Bademan.
        p. ; cm.
    ISBN 978-1-930538-89-4
1. Intensive care nursing--Miscellanea. I. Sigma Theta Tau International. II. Title.
    [DNLM: 1. Critical Care--Almanacs. 2. Nursing Care--Almanacs. WY 154 B133d 2010]
    RT120.I5B33 2010
    616.02'8--dc22
                                                2009046377
First Printing, 2009

Publisher: Renee Wilmeth   Copy Editor: Jacqueline Tiery
Acquisitions Editor: Cover Designer: Gary Adair
    Cynthia Saver, RN, MS   Interior Design and Page
Editorial Coordinator: Paula Jeffers   Composition: Rebecca Batchelor
Development Editor: Carla Hall

Dedication

To all the women and men of acute and critical care nursing whose tireless efforts, genuine compassion, and enduring commitment to their chosen profession has touched the lives of countless patients, families, and colleagues. Know that the work you do is deeply meaningful and appreciated by those you serve.

–Eileen Gallen Bademan

Acknowledgements

Sincere thanks to all who so eagerly and willingly contributed to this project. Thanks also to Cindy Saver and the folks at Sigma Theta Tau International for all their help and support. It was truly an honor compiling this daybook. Special thanks to the American Association of Critical-Care Nurses (AACN) for their assistance in content development and to Mary Jo Grap for the many "clinical pearls" she compiled for the *American Journal of Critical Care,* some of which are shared throughout the book.

–Eileen Gallen Bademan

About the Author

Eileen Gallen Bademan, BSN, RN, has been in nursing for more than 20 years, beginning in acute care at the Hospital of the University of Pennsylvania and shifting to critical care at Williamsport Hospital and Medical Center in the intensive care unit. In the late 1990s, she entered the publishing world, first as clinical manager for drug information products at Lippincott, Williams & Wilkins, then most recently as the editorial manager for *American Nurse Today*—the official journal of the American Nurses Association. Eileen now lives in Yardley, Pennsylvania, with her husband Steve, their five children—Nicole, Sarah, Lauren, Steven, and Kate—and their dog, Tink.

Table of Contents

Foreword

A popular soft drink once distinguished itself as "the pause that refreshes." Nurses should be known for our well-honed ability to take a refreshing pause. Our chosen work, to paraphrase nurse researcher and scholar, Virginia Henderson, is to support individuals in activities that contribute to health, to the regaining of health, or to achieving a peaceful death. Whenever we forego that short pause to reflect and refocus on the meaning of our work, we deplete our emotional and physical reserves and diminish our indispensable contribution to the life and death of fellow human beings.

Nurses in high acuity and critical care should be among the most skillful and practiced in the art of refreshing pauses, because we are singularly vulnerable. We care for the sickest patients and their families, wherever they may be: always in critical care and progressive care units of hospitals, and increasingly, often in medical-surgical units; we are also present on-scene after accidents, on battlefields, in transport vehicles, in skilled care facilities, and in homes. We are even in tele-ICUs where we expertly guide the care of patients hundreds and thousands of miles away.

The Honor Society of Nursing, Sigma Theta Tau International (STTI), invited the American Association of Critical-Care Nurses (AACN) to collaborate in developing the first daybook specifically for clinical nurses. AACN welcomed this invitation to collaborate on the development of this unique resource that prompts and prods us in mastering the art of the pause—the pause that will refresh us, renew us, and support us in our critical work.

This book is uniquely AACN. Many of the daily affirmations and brief topical essays are selected from the messages of AACN presidents. Typical of high acuity and critical care nurses, the words of AACN presidents challenge and inspire. They hug and they prod. Their words encourage and renew, drawing from the deep well of experience gained from life in the community of their chosen professional association. Clinical pearls, many of them from the *American Journal of Critical Care*, draw closure to each month and remind us of the technical realities of our work.

Energized by its refreshing pauses, *A Daybook for Critical Care Nurses* will help us embrace timeless issues that challenge and empower us—issues like following the evidence-based path of best practices, making tough decisions with confidence and compassion, and advocating for the vulnerable, who may be patients, families, or even colleagues. As we reflect on these issues, we will find renewed strength in nursing's honored tradition and share in the wisdom of our colleagues.

Take care of yourself, and help others do the same.

—Beth Hammer, RN, MSN, APN-BC
2009-2010 President,
American Association of Critical-Care Nurses

—Maria Shirey, RN, PhD, MBA, NEA-BC, FACHE
2009-2011 Chair, AACN Certification Corporation

Introduction

Ask any group of nurses why they chose nursing as their profession, and chances are pretty good no one will answer, "For fame, fortune, and glory." As a matter of fact, I believe most would answer, "Because I want to help people." After all, isn't that at the core of what we do? We help people through their acute and critical illnesses; we help their families understand what is happening; we help our colleagues through mentoring, understanding, and "chipping in" when they are having a difficult day; and we help others through our knowledge, expertise, compassion, and commitment. But what do *you* do to help *yourself*? It is easy to put ourselves on the back burner after we have cared for everyone else—but we all know, in the end, we have robbed ourselves of the precious moment of renewal. And renewal can literally take just a moment. A moment for you! Time to reflect, be inspired, stimulated, identify with the words of others, and learn something new about ourselves.

A Daybook for Critical Care Nurses is the first daybook for specialty nurses. Developed in collaboration with the American Association of Critical-Care Nurses, this book can be your personal tool—a living journal, if you will. Each month begins with a short essay addressing one of the many important topics you face every day in your practice. Then, each day of the month has a daily inspiration, a personal thought or encouragement, a humorous glimpse at ourselves, a message of hope or motivation, or a recognition of the important work you do. Use the space provided below each entry to journal. It's amazing how the simple act of writing your thoughts on paper releases new energies and ideas. Then, take the time to look back on what you have written. You may be surprised at what you learn about yourself. Share some of your favorite quotes with your co-workers—or write them on a sticky note and put it on the mirror in the staff bathroom or on one of the computer terminals at the nurse's station. Chances are someone else may feel as inspired as you do. Remind yourself everyday of the great work you do and the invaluable impact you have on your patients, their families, your colleagues, and your community, as you continue to do what nurses do best—helping others.

—Eileen Gallen Bademan

Compassion

As critical care nurses, our contribution of compassion is inseparable from being fully present. Compassion is more than being nice, and it's more than being knowledgeable and competent. It is the way we truly live inside someone else's skin—treating patients with dignity, caring about them as people, showing concern for their worries, spending time with them, collaborating to care for them, and focusing on their special needs—including their culture, race, and spiritual beliefs.

Today, there is so much that derails our best intentions of being compassionate. Yet sustaining compassion is essential for nurses to survive—and thrive. It is the quality that uniquely defines nurses' contributions to health care.

Patients and families have everything to gain from our compassionate competence; it turns the most horrific illnesses into life-changing experiences, bringing families closer and uncovering resources that they themselves seldom knew they had. The healing energy of our compassion often drives that transformation. Compassion allows us to treat people with dignity, be fully present so we can uncover their unique needs, and invest in meeting those needs. Compassion means we care enough about people and their worries that we rally our colleagues to offer our best chance for a cure or for a peaceful death.

Compassion that flows from us must come back to us. We have chosen a tough profession, one where our shared contributions are needed today perhaps more than ever. We reaffirm our choice of becoming a nurse and prevent our compassion from waning when we are supported in talking safely about our feelings, needs, and fears. When we can use our talents to connect, to care and to truly make a difference, we are nourished in return. We receive the satisfaction that flows from making a critical illness the best experience it can be for a patient and family.

–*Kathy McCauley, RN, PhD, BC, FAAN, FAHA*

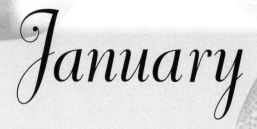

January

January 1

"The cool air rushes in and the world is quieted by a blanket of dancing snowflakes, a warm fire, the scent of spruce and cinnamon is in the air. January is a time of new beginnings, promises, and crisp change. It's a chance for resolution and tenacity. What will this new year bring for you, an extraordinary nurse?"

–Sharon Hudacek, RN, EdD
From A Daybook for Nurses: Making a Difference Each Day

January 2

"Although we may not know it, we are most likely heroes in our daily lives. Nurses offer an extraordinary gift—caring for others at the most vulnerable times in their lives."

–Debbie Brinker, RN, MSN, CCRN, CCNS

January 3

"Peace is not the absence of pain. Peace is a certainty of living life
for a worthy purpose, knowing that we are becoming a better
person and touching the lives of others every day."

–Sharon M. Weinstein, MS, RN, CRNI, FAAN
From B is for Balance

January 4

"I remember a patient in the CCU who was on an intra-aortic
balloon pump for an inordinate amount of time. I would share a
soda with him each night I worked, and we'd talk a little about his
feelings. After his death, I realized that the best gift I had given
him wasn't all the technical care…it was spending those few
minutes with him—the gift of time."

–Cynthia Saver, RN, MS

JANUARY 5

"When talking and listening, make sure your intent is to discover
and understand, not to persuade."

—Denise Thornby, RN, MS

JANUARY 6

"The gift we can offer each other is so simple a thing as hope."

—Daniel Berrigan

JANUARY 7

"Nurses are a hospital's most precious resource and the one that
is in shortest supply. Would you expect a precious resource to go
chasing after urinals and linens?"

—Dorrie Fontaine, RN, DNSc, FAAN

JANUARY 8

"Time is the coin of your life. It is the only coin you have, and only you can determine how it will be spent. Be careful, lest you let other people spend it for you."

–Carl Sandburg

JANUARY 9

"Compassion is the sometimes-fatal capacity for feeling what it's like to live inside somebody else's skin. It is the knowledge that there can never be any peace and joy for me until there is peace and joy finally for you too."

–Frederick Buechner

JANUARY 10

"Compassion makes an impersonal health care system personal and
turns the worst day of someone's life into the best day it can be."

—Kathy McCauley, RN, PhD, BC, FAAN, FAHA

JANUARY 11

"Always role model collaboration and partnerships.
Guide newer staff in developing their collaborative skills.
Influence others by your actions."

—Denise Thornby, RN, MS

January 12

"Take the time to truly understand one another. Do not dismiss
someone who shares a different perspective than you,
because the most valuable learning often comes from
uncomfortable situations."

–Michael L. Williams, RN, MSN, CCRN

January 13

"As a nurse in the intensive care unit, our eyes are the first that
family members look into for the hope they seek that everything
will be OK."

–James Stovall, BSN, RN

JANUARY 14

"Awareness comes not only from being in touch with values and talents but, perhaps more importantly, gaining significance through willingness to take the risk of questioning yourself and being open to external input."

—Nancy Dickenson-Hazard, RN, MSN, FAAN
From Ready, Set, Go Lead!

JANUARY 15

"What you cannot turn to good, you must make as little bad as you can."

—Sir Thomas More

January 16

"Asking questions is a direct path to exploring, growing, learning."
—*Mary Fran Tracy, RN, PhD, CCNS, CCRN, FAAN*

January 17

"When we cannot or do not pay attention, clearing the clutter from the moment, we create untold hazards that can endanger us and others."
—*Dave Hanson, RN, MSN, CCRN, CNS*

January 18

"Treat yourself healthfully…You must provide the best for yourself before it's available to others."
—*Mary Anne Radmacher*

January 19

"When I was a new graduate, I entered the PICU with five peers—all of us with great trepidation at the task ahead of us. Twelve years later, I returned to the same unit as manager of some of the same nurses I'd worked with previously. At the moment I accepted the job, I made a commitment to always remember how it feels to be a new graduate in critical care and to lend a welcoming hand to students and new nurses. Not necessarily to be a hero, but to do the right thing as an advocate for patients first, then for nurses."

—Debbie Brinker, RN, MSN, CCRN, CCNS

January 20

"With purpose comes all kinds of possibilities for taking confident actions that matter to our patients."

—Caryl Goodyear-Bruch, RN, PhD, CCRN

JANUARY 21

"Nursing engages in a life-death journey, participates in birthing-living-suffering-playing-loving-dying as the very fabric of human existence. The moral and visionary compass for my journey comes not from the head but from the heart."

–Jean Watson, PhD, RN, AHN-BC, FAAN
From Conversations with Leaders

JANUARY 22

"Life is not a path of coincidence, happenstance, and luck, but rather an unexplainable, meticulously charted course for one to touch the lives of others and make a difference in the world."

–Barbara Dillinham, MSc

January 23

"Spend time with those who nourish you, who empower you to be the best you can be—those who help you make the right choices in your life."

–Denise Thornby, RN, MS

January 24

"Being present is the fuel that feeds our contribution and our professionalism. It expands our vast repertoire of knowledge, solidifies our credibility, and gives us the most satisfaction."

–Kathy McCauley, RN, PhD, BC, FAAN, FAHA

JANUARY 25

"Without dialogue around challenges, nothing at work will
ever change."

—Connie Barden, RN, MSN, CCNS, CCRN

JANUARY 26

"For me, rising above means seeking a new level of consciousness
to objectively and truthfully see current reality for what it is—and
what it is not."

—Dorrie Fontaine, RN, DNSc, FAAN

JANUARY 27

"If nurses have a shared passion, it is clearly our passion to care.
We have cornered the market on caring for others. This is our calling. This is our journey. This is our inextinguishable inner fire."

—Michael L. Williams, RN, MSN, CCRN

January 28

"Clinical scholarship is about inquiry and implies a willingness to scrutinize our practice, even if it means challenging the theories and procedures that we learned and practice. It's looking for a different and better way to nurse and refusing to accept anything just because that's the way in which it always has been done."

–Melanie Dreher, PhD, RN, FAAN

January 29

"To be empathetic, you also must be vulnerable and courageous. You risk emotional vulnerability when truly being present with another."

–Marjorie Schaffer, RN, BA, MS, PhD, and
Linda Norlander, RN, BSN, MS
From Being Present: A Nurse's Resource for
End-of-Life Communication

JANUARY 30

"Creativity is not some mystical power bestowed on a chosen few.
We all have it—just take a look at any group of children and
witness their wonder, curiosity, and boldness."

—Nancy Dickenson-Hazard, RN, MSN, FAAN
From Ready, Set, Go Lead!

JANUARY 31

CLINICAL PEARL

Do you know how to prepare families for withdrawal of life support from their loved one? Specific messages include the following:

- Uncertainty concerning time of death
- Reassurance that nursing care will continue
- Symptom management is the priority
- Privacy will be provided
- General signs: breathing pattern changes, skin color
  changes, muscle spasms
- Families may choose to stay or leave at any time
- Permission given to touch, talk to the patient, or
  assist with care

Kirchhoff, K., Palzkill, J., Kowalkowski, J., Mork, A., Gretarsdottir, E.
(2008). Preparing Families of Intensive Care Patients for Withdrawal
of Life Support: A Pilot Study. American Journal of Critical Care,
17(2), 113-121.

Making Better Decisions

Almost daily, we must decide whether to take the "high road" or the "low road" when confronted with difficult situations. By taking the high road, we choose to exercise positive influence, an act that requires courage and helps us focus others and ourselves on the future. Taking the low road, on the other hand, is never a fulfilling journey. It drains you of needed energy.

When we consistently take the high road, we truly become leaders within our profession. We can influence others to pause at the crossroads and think a little harder before they choose their route. We can help them find the courage to take the high road when faced with challenging situations.

Here are some travel tips to help you on your journey through the day:

- Encourage colleagues to speak directly to one another if there is an issue or concern regarding their practice.

- Be truthful and honest, yet deliver your message clearly, giving others a chance to share their side of the story.

- Help others learn from their mistakes.

- Acknowledge the "baby steps" of improvement we all make when learning a new skill.

- Use inquiry to better understand a situation and avoid assumptions and judgments.

- Always strive for excellence, while accepting that perfectionism is in the mind of the beholder and never completely achievable.

- Let the values of respect, trustworthiness, dignity, and courage guide your actions.

The road you choose tells the world a great deal about you, your courage, and your values. The high road is proactive and future-focused. When you take the high road, you are part of the solution.

–Denise Thornby, RN, MS

February

February 1

"Don't wait for something big to occur. Start where you are,
with what you have, and that will always lead you into
something greater."

—Mary Mannin Morrissey

February 2

"Having a team we can count on is essential to us being able to do
our best for patients. Treating them with dignity and working with
them, their families, and our colleagues to achieve their wishes are
privileges we honor and share with one another."

—Caryl Goodyear-Bruch, RN, PhD, CCRN

FEBRUARY 3

"Nurses are what make or break the health systems and the health status of people. Every day, a multitude of nurses leads a multitude of patients to well-being."

—Nancy Dickenson-Hazard, RN, MSN, FAAN

FEBRUARY 4

"One's destination is never a place, but rather, a new way of looking at things."

—Henry Miller

FEBRUARY 5

"Read the nursing articles in your journals for true understanding, not simply to earn CE credits."

—Michael L. Williams, RN, MSN, CCRN

February 6

"Wherever we care for critically ill patients and their families—
ICUs, step-down units, high-acuity med-surg units, emergency
departments—nurses form part of an ensemble cast delivering
timeless messages as part of our everyday work."

–Dorrie Fontaine, RN, DNSc, FAAN

February 7

"Take a leadership role in building bridges between team members,
units, and departments, all in the name of doing what is in the best
interest of patients."

–Denise Thornby, RN, MS

February 8

"My 22-year-old patient died. He lived many years beyond what was expected for his condition. His elderly father, who had been so vigilant during his son's ICU stay, had finally gone home to take a rest. I had to call him to come back. Upon arriving to the unit, the father hugged me hard and tearfully thanked me for the care I gave to his son. Then we both went into the room to say goodbye."

—Eileen Gallen Bademan, RN, BSN

February 9

"True collaboration is more than coordination and cooperation. It demonstrates shared objectives and different skill sets coupled with heartfelt commitment."

—Mary Fran Tracy, RN, PhD, CCNS, CCRN, FAAN

February 10

"When you fail to use the power you have by virtue of your position, your expertise, or your access to information, you miss opportunities for yourself, your patients, and your profession."

—Eleanor Sullivan, RN, PhD

February 11

"Nurses usually excel at ethically driven clinical practice.
No wonder the public repeatedly identifies us as the profession
most trusted to act honestly and ethically."

—Kathy McCauley, RN, PhD, BC, FAAN, FAHA

February 12

"A ringing call bell light in the ICU means transfer orders
are on the way."

—James Stovall, BSN, RN

February 13

"If I'm not uncomfortable, I'm not growing."

—Nancy C. Molter, RN, MN, PhD

February 14

"Fear and resignation are the enemies of inspired work that makes
us feel enlivened by what we do."

—Connie Barden, RN, MSN, CCNS, CCRN

February 15

"In my experience, most critical care nurses want to support new graduates. I believe all of us are accountable to confront it [detrimental behavior] when we see it. Our legacy of 'eating our young' or 'putting them through their paces' must stop with us. If we do not put an end to this, it will destroy us."

—Denise Thornby, RN, MS

February 16

"Our work relies on relationships—establishing, sustaining, and building them. We need each other, and our patients need us to work together."

—Caryl Goodyear-Bruch, RN, PhD, CCRN

February 17

"Work with men in nursing to model effective communication across genders. Give us directions, even when we may forget to ask for them! It's the work that matters, not the gender of the provider!"

–Michael L. Williams, RN, MSN, CCRN

February 18

"Ultimate patient care doesn't happen automatically when nurses ask, think, investigate, and define their practice. Ultimate care happens when, driven by our purpose, research enhances the experience and judgment that come from years of nursing."

–Connie Barden, RN, MSN, CCNS, CCRN

February 19

"We have the choice of allowing circumstances to control us or being a catalyst for change by expressing and acting on our values."

—Nancy Dickenson-Hazard RN, MSN, FAAN
From Ready, Set, Go Lead!

February 20

"The ICU is where 'Protect and Serve' meets 'It Takes A Village.'"

—Sonya Holder, ADN, RN, CCRN

February 21

"To change and to change for the better are two different things."

—German Proverb

February 22

"In our tireless work caring for others, we often forget to care for ourselves. We must make time for deliberate, focused renewal. Let's commit that we will take this time for ourselves so that we can be faithful to those for whom we care."

–Michael L. Williams, RN, MSN, CCRN

February 23

"I remind myself to focus on what I have that is good and right in my life, which always begins the momentum needed to move me ahead."

–June Kasiak-Gambla
From A Daybook for Nurses: Making a Difference Each Day

February 24

"We knew coming into this work of critical care that the challenges
would be great and many. We also knew that the rewards would
be rich and meaningful. In fact, that's what attracted many of us.
It takes a special breed of person to aspire to this demanding
profession."

—Denise Thornby, RN, MS

February 25

"The only very interesting answers are those which destroy the
questions."

—Susan Sontag

February 26

"I marvel at how confidence from a respected stranger can be as
energizing as that of a trusted friend."

–Dorrie Fontaine, RN, DNSc, FAAN

February 27

"Like any journey, ours has an origin and a destination. As we forge
our path, we will become open to new ideas, to new strategies for
care, to seeing ourselves in new ways. There will be new things to
observe and understand, new lessons to learn, and new challenges
to our beliefs and skills."

–Michael L. Williams, RN, MSN, CCRN

FEBRUARY 28

CLINICAL PEARL

Endotracheal tube cuff pressure is often estimated by palpating the pilot balloon, but studies show this technique is inaccurate, with less than one-third of the pressures within therapeutic range.

Sole, M.L., Aragon Penoyer, D., Su, X., Jimenez, E., Kalita, S.J., Poalillo, E., et al. (2009). Assessment of Endotracheal Cuff Pressure by Continuous Monitoring: A Pilot Study. American Journal of Critical Care, *18(2), 133-143.*

FEBRUARY 29

(FOR LEAP OR INTERCALARY YEARS)

"I will never forget the critical care nurses who 'raised' me in the specialty. I can still picture them more than 30 years later. We must always take novice colleagues under our wings to teach them the true art and science of acute and critical care."

–Melissa A. Fitzpatrick, RN, MSN

BUILDING BETTER COLLABORATIVE PARTNERS

True collaboration is how we become full partners. And, to be full partners we must be willing to know what others do. True collaboration means dialogue where everyone learns and comes together to a greater truth, all to the benefit of patients and their families. True collaboration holds each person accountable for presenting an honest and thorough perspective, supported by evidence that helps to consider alternatives.

Following are some ways you can cultivate collaboration:

- Listen closely to the perspectives of others; they will help you to recognize blind spots in your own thinking.

- Engage in dialogue. When talking and listening with others, make sure your intent is to discover and understand, not to persuade.

- Getting to know those with whom you wish to collaborate will make finding a common ground easier.

- Acknowledge the strengths and contributions that other team members bring to the care of patients.

- Always model by your actions.

- Pay close attention to group dynamics. Often, the root of conflict starts when there are misperceptions about the intent behind a breach in process.

- Find opportunities to learn with other members of the interdisciplinary team.

- Celebrate your successes together.

- Lastly, and most importantly, keep your eye on the goal of collaboration.

We all must use our skills to collaborate with other disciplines that join us in caring for the critically ill. By joining together and creating a shared vision of a health care system driven by the needs of patients, all caregivers can make their optimal contribution.

–Denise Thornby, RN, MS, & Kathy McCauley, RN, PhD, BC, FAAN, FAHA

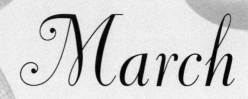

March

March 1

"I don't need to convince you that your contribution to patients, health care, and society is invaluable. Please take the time to reflect about these experiences because they represent the real reasons we became nurses."

–Kathy McCauley, RN, PhD, BC, FAAN, FAHA

March 2

"Crucial conversations can help us learn to dialogue with genuine intention that gets positive results. A crucial conversation involves two or more people when the stakes are high, opinions vary, and emotions run strong."

–Dorrie Fontaine, RN, DNSc, FAAN

March 3

"In the ICU we live by a certain code:
If they bleed, stop it.
If they are not breathing, tube them.
If their heart stops, shock it.
And if they can push the call light, transfer them."

—James Stovall, BSN, RN

March 4

"Learning to appreciate others' perspectives takes time and soul searching. We must first understand ourselves to appreciate differences in others."

—Michael L. Williams, RN, MSN, CCRN

March 5

"Nurses save lives. Nurses rescue patients. Nurses do for others what they can't do for themselves. We take patients from crisis to resolution."

–Connie Barden, RN, MSN, CCNS, CCRN

March 6

"Just as the ocean waves continually shape the landscape by moving the sand, one grain at a time, critical care nurses can make a difference in health care, one life at a time."

–Denise Thornby, RN, MS

March 7

"Success is all about using and getting used, and knowing when both are happening."

–Susan Sherman, RN, MA
From Conversations with Leaders

March 8

"Through grace, we add a measure of healing by sharing a human connection with the patient as a person. A comfortable relationship is in itself a reassuring action."

—Alan Briskin and Jan Boller
From Daily Miracles

March 9

"To become fully competent, we must understand, hone, recognize, and celebrate it. But above all, we must demand it."

—Kathy McCauley, RN, PhD, BC, FAAN, FAHA

MARCH 10

"Health care is a team sport—an extreme sport, really. If we are
not competent as a team, we suffer, and our patients
and families suffer."

—Debbie Brinker, RN, MSN, CCRN, CCNS

MARCH 11

"A wise person once said, 'If we always agree on everything,
then one of us is unnecessary.'"

—Anonymous

March 12

"Care about your patient like you would care about
your own loved one."

–Susanne Thees, RN

March 13

"Acknowledge the strengths and contributions that others bring to
the care of critically ill patients or the outcomes the team achieves.
Acknowledging the value of their contributions will go a long way
toward making everyone feel valued."

–Denise Thornby, RN, MS

March 14

"Purpose is the result you want to create…it is where your values
and talents make a solid connection to everyday actions."

–Nancy Dickenson-Hazard, RN, MSN, FAAN
From Ready, Set, Go Lead!

March 15

"You are not an expert simply because you follow physicians' orders
or care about your patients. You should be revered for talents such
as analytical thinking, inquiry, and observation skills; patient ad-
vocacy expertise; and the sound clinical judgment required daily at
the bedside to prevent catastrophe, complications, and even death."

–Connie Barden, RN, MSN, CCNS, CCRN

March 16

"Remember what it was like to be a new graduate. We need you to create an atmosphere of caring for and about us as we begin our professional careers."

—Aurora Hernandez, RN

March 17

"Develop your leadership skills, but remember that leadership isn't a job or a title. Leaders influence people and situations to bring about transforming change."

—From A Daybook for Nurse Leaders and Mentors

March 18

"Why does the altitude of your rear control the timing of your pump alarm?"

—Sonya Holder, ADN, RN, CCRN

March 19

"Early in my career, my first clinical nurse specialist wrote
me a note to congratulate me on how I handled a particularly
challenging situation. That note, which I still have, works wonders
for me when I re-read it on a 'down' day. I keep it with other
affirming notes and cards that keep me focused on my journey of
rediscovery—a journey where I'm looking in and finding myself,
reaching out, and helping others."

—Michael L. Williams, RN, MSN, CCRN

March 20

"Be conscious of effective interpersonal communication skills. Use
these to communicate not only your perspective, but also your
respect for the individual with whom you are communicating."

—Denise Thornby, RN, MS

March 21

"Remember the many times your presence made something wonderful happen for a patient, a family, a new nurse, an experienced nurse nearing the end of his or her career. Ask yourself how you will use this inspiration to stay in the game."

–Kathy McCauley, RN, PhD, BC, FAAN, FAHA

March 22

"Every life is significant and every death should be with dignity."

–Lisa Bonsall, RN, MSN, CRNP

March 23

"Miracles come when you least expect them."

–Susanne Thees, RN

MARCH 24

"I invite you to raise your own bar and take the step to becoming the powerful force that can create a new future. Tomorrow is in our hands. And it is the voices and actions of thousands of critical care nurses boldly declaring a new vision for health care and a new day for nurses that will create that new tomorrow."

—Connie Barden, RN, MSN, CCRN

MARCH 25

"Give yourself positive feedback when you're doing a good job."

—Michael L. Williams, RN, MSN, CCRN

March 26

"I believe that one of nursing's most significant contributions to health care is the never-ending vigilance to ensure safe passage of patients through the system."

—Denise Thornby, RN, MS

March 27

"Empowerment is risky, but without risk, there is no creativity or learning."

—Nancy Dickenson-Hazard, RN, MSN, FAAN
From Ready, Set, Go Lead!

MARCH 28

"In your thirst for knowledge, be sure not to drown
in all the information."

–Anthony J. D'Angelo

MARCH 29

"Like so many nursing interventions, being creative has many
forms. Simple things like listening and sensing something is wrong
can be creative because it is a strategy for reaching deeper and
finding out what is really happening."

–Sharon Hudacek, RN, EdD
From Making a Difference: Stories From the Point of Care, Volume I

MARCH 30

"Do not do unto others as you expect they should do unto you. Their tastes may not be the same."

—George Bernard Shaw

MARCH 31

CLINICAL PEARL

Malnutrition has negative effects on the critically ill. National guidelines for nutrition recommend the following:

- Initiate enteral nutrition within 24 to 48 hours after ICU admission.

- If possible, use postpyloric nutrition based on a trend toward reducing infectious complications.

- Elevate the head of the patient's bed to 45° during enteral feeding, or, if contraindicated, elevate as high as possible.

O'Meara, D., Mireles-Cabodevila, E., Frame, F., Hummell, A.C., Hammel, J., Dweik, R.A.,et al. (2008). Evaluation of Delivery of Enteral Nutrition in Critically Ill Patients Receiving Mechanical Ventilation. American Journal of Critical Care, *17(1), 53-61.*

EVIDENCE-BASED PRACTICE

Ultimate patient care doesn't happen automatically when nurses ask, think, investigate, and define their practice. Ultimate care happens when, driven by our purpose, research enhances the experience and judgment that come from years of nursing. Many nurses have the misconception that asking questions, looking for answers, and incorporating the answers into practice as the purview of academic faculty, not of nurses in clinical practice. Actually, nobody is better suited to participate in clinical inquiry and drive the discovery of answers than nurses at the bedside. Clinical nurses must accept the responsibility to question, study, and define the care we give. Critical care changes at a rapid pace, so nursing practice must be based on available evidence and research. This cannot be optional. Evidence cannot be used when convenient and ignored when taxing or unfamiliar.

The expertise gained during years of clinical practice is certainly another basic element of a mature and evolving practice. But experience alone is not a sufficient teacher. Indeed, care based solely on tradition or dated information is dangerous as it threatens patients and their outcomes.

It is essential to re-engage our shared commitment to exceptional care by embracing the findings of research and incorporating them into daily practice. Anything less than this level of excellence diminishes our optimal contribution to patient care and dampens the spirit that inspires our work.

Combining decades of experience with the results of inquiry creates truly exceptional care. Besides creating incomparable outcomes for patients, families, and nurses, you'll re-invent the standard by which you practice and re-engage the spirit of those with whom you work. An environment steeped in inquisitiveness and excitement about practice is like a magnet. Nurses clamor to work there. Embrace the opportunity to create that environment.

–Connie Barden, RN, MSN, CCNS, CCRN

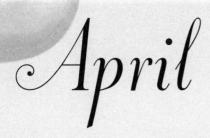

April

April 1

"The pain in your feet at the end of your shift is directly related to the number of times you forgot why you went to the supply cart."

—Sonya Holder, ADN, RN, CCRN

April 2

"Every day you make choices about how to act or respond. Through these acts, you have the power to positively influence."

—Denise Thornby, RN, MS

April 3

"Review your efforts and reframe them when a particularly challenging case comes your way. A patient's peaceful and dignified death is often a triumph, not a failure."

—Michael L. Williams, RN, MSN, CCRN

April 4

"Moments of daily renewal are like seeds that sprout and burrow deep into the soil of our lives as a free and irrepressible melody of hope. Such moments are as close as a shaft of sunlight breaking through the morning mist, or a red-tailed hawk serenely catching an updraft and then allowing itself to be launched across the vast expanses of the sky. Such magic at only the price of our attention! No need to grasp greedily at such moments: They come upon us naturally—yes, repeatedly—in the utter simplicity and fullness of life. There is more than enough for us all."

—The Monks of New Skete

April 5

"A 'No' uttered from deepest conviction is better and greater than a 'Yes' merely uttered to please, or what is worse, to avoid trouble."

—Mohandas K. Gandhi

April 6

"It isn't adversity that defeats people. People are defeated by their inability to see how to change the way things are."

—Connie Barden, RN, MSN, CCNS, CCRN

April 7

"Show me a dry bag of levophed and I'll show you a nurse in ventricular tachycarda."

—Sonya Holder, ADN, RN, CCRN

April 8

"When fear stops us, it means we have made it our master when our true masters ought to be our knowledge, skills, and abilities."

—Caryl Goodyear-Bruch, RN, PhD, CCRN

April 9

"At the end of a long and busy shift in the ICU, have you ever looked back and realized with satisfaction that 'because I was here today,' something remarkable happened? Your presence, your actions, made the critical difference in achieving a positive outcome."

—Kathy McCauley, RN, PhD, BC, FAAN, FAHA

April 10

"Nurses must be as proficient in communication skills as
they are in clinical skills."

−AACN Standards for Establishing and Sustaining
Healthy Work Environments: A Journey to Excellence

April 11

"Although each of us is on a personal journey, we cannot forget
that our colleagues are, too. None of us is on this journey alone.
We must draw from the strengths of our colleagues and value these
strengths as the precious gifts that they are."

−Michael L. Williams, RN, MSN, CCRN

April 12

"True collaboration is based on openness to one another's unique skills and perspectives, which will be revealed only through skilled communication."

—Mary Fran Tracy, RN, PhD, CCNS, CCRN, FAAN

April 13

"An insight has the capacity to take something that you know in your head and make you feel it in your gut."

—Phil Dusenberry

April 14

"Situations that are genuinely uncontrollable cannot be changed. We either need to remove them or put them in perspective so they don't deplete our energy and produce diminished or empty returns."

—Dave Hanson, RN, MSN, CCRN, CNS

April 15

"You have the ability and opportunity to influence your daily life.
You also have the ability and opportunity to make a difference in
the lives of others, which is the greatest achievement of all."

—Denise Thornby, RN, MS

April 16

"We can't genuinely engage in our work when we aren't meaning-
fully recognized and respected for our values and for our contributions to our patients, our unit, and our organization."

—Debbie Brinker, RN, MSN, CCRN, CCNS

April 17

"Always do right—this will gratify some and astonish the rest."
—Mark Twain

April 18

"We must be certain that our colleagues know how vital nurses are to patient outcomes and why hospitals cannot afford to let nursing care be anything but the best."
—Connie Barden, RN, MSN, CCNS, CCRN

APRIL 19

"Leaders earn and respect the trust of others, in part by showing
they know the difference between what may be important
and what is truly urgent."

–Caryl Goodyear-Bruch, RN, PhD, CCRN

APRIL 20

"We must never lose sight of how critical it is to preserve
what makes each of us a nurse."

–Kim Doherty
From A Daybook for Nurses: Making a Difference Each Day

APRIL 21

"We don't see things as they are; we see them as we are."

–Anaïs Nin

APRIL 22

"The Latin words engraved on an iron gate at the University of
Pennsylvania sum up nursing for me: 'We will find a way,
or we will make a way.'"

–Kathy McCauley, RN, PhD, BC, FAAN, FAHA

APRIL 23

"To build teams within critical care that attract and retain the best
of the best, we must be accountable for having the skills necessary
to confront our coworkers, to coach them in gaining effective interpersonal skills, and to support them in their efforts to develop
the skills of emotional intelligence."

–Denise Thornby, RN, MS

April 24

"Remember that critical care nurses offer something more powerful than all the new drugs and latest medical technology—our personal connection with our patients in knowing what they need and how to provide that all powerful healing effect of simply caring."

–Denise Thornby, RN, MS

April 25

"Why do we hesitate to use our power and influence? Using influence means taking risks. This requires being confident about the value of our knowledge and perspective. It means becoming visible and engaged, perhaps leaving our comfort zone."

–Mary Fran Tracy, RN, PhD, CCNS, CCRN, FAAN

April 26

"Communication is a fundamental priority we must reclaim
in support of our core values of patients and families,
safety and reliability."

—Dave Hanson, RN, MSN, CCRN, CNS

April 27

"Nurse are cost effective. We save money while keeping patients
safe. To accomplish this requires a solid professional education,
astute clinical reasoning, and expert clinical thinking."

Caryl Goodyear-Bruch, RN, PhD, CCRN

April 28

"Resignation will always whisper that speaking up won't
make a difference. I truly believe, however, that it is the
only thing that will."

—Connie Barden, RN, MSN, CCRN

April 29

"As critical care nurses, our individual spirits and our collective
code of ethics compel us to be engaged. Few occupations can
afford people who are not engaged. But health care is
downright dangerous when we are not."

–Debbie Brinker, RN, MSN, CCNS, CCRN

April 30

Clinical Pearl

One study found that when the cuff pressure was maintained
below 20 cm H_2O, the risk for ventilator-associated
pneumonia was four times higher.

*Sole, M.L., Aragon Penoyer, D., Su, X., Jimenez, E., Kalita, S.J.,
Poalillo, E., et al. (2009). Assessment of Endotracheal Cuff Pressure by
Continuous Monitoring: A Pilot Study.* American Journal of
Critical Care, *18(2), 133-143.*

Being a Critical Care Nurse

As a critical care nurse, we have the ability to positively influence the lives of so many people with our decisions and actions. It is not the just the lives of our patient's we touch, but that of their families and others in their lives.

We meet our patients and their families at the worst possible time in their lives. We expect the families to know and follow the rules, and to leave after only of a few minutes of visitation, leaving their loved one's life in the hands of complete strangers. A critical care nurse is one who, with knowledge and talent, can save the lives of their patients while managing the many critical and delicate situations that arise.

However, we must realize that we are not always able to save everyone. I remember a nurse telling me one day, "This is so hard. The patient is dying and there is nothing I can do, yet his family keeps thanking me for everything I have done." These are the times where it is all about supporting the family. The critical care nurse is the one who touches the heart of the family through their acts of kindness, compassion, encouragement, and understanding—even if the patient passes away.

We help save the lives of others. Some of our patients sustain non-survivable injuries and their families are faced with making the decision of having their loved one become an organ donor. Critical care nurses, through their relationships with the families, can help explain the process and the benefits of such a decision. Critical care nurses serve not only as their patient's advocate, but also as an advocate for others.

Being a critical care nurse is extremely fulfilling. We touch many lives, bond with many families, and make many new friendships. And the best reward is when our patient's come back to us—for a visit!

–Charles Reed, MSN, RN, CNRN

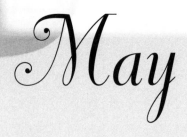

May

May 1

"Never give up on yourself. When I started in the CCU as a new grad, we were in the midst of yet another nursing shortage, and I was 'team leading' before I had my ECG course. I went home and cried after my first few codes, convinced I wasn't up for the job. But you know what? I hung in there and little by little—with the help of some wonderful nurse mentors—eventually felt confident with codes and went on to become a preceptor for other 'newbies.'"

–Cynthia Saver, RN, MS

May 2

"Being empathetic is hard to teach. Empathy must be felt, lived, and experienced, and that takes many nursing episodes to learn."

–Sharon Hudacek, RN, EdD
From Making a Difference: Stories From the Point of Care, Volume I

MAY 3

"If we are to truly create environments where every critical care nurse can make his or her optimal contribution, all of us must be skilled in interpersonal relationships and have a high degree of emotional intelligence."

–Denise Thornby, RN, MS

MAY 4

"Nurses' relationships with patients are roadmaps for the best care because they grow from being fully present. Nurses know how to overcome barriers to understanding what a patient feels and needs in the moment. We overcome those barriers because of presence that is anchored not only in emotion, but also in knowledge."

–Kathy McCauley, RN, PhD, BC, FAAN, FAHA

May 5

"It is worth striving to get the right relationships between yourself and others, between yourself and your work, and between yourself and something larger than yourself. If you get these relationships right, a sense of purpose and meaning will emerge."

–Jonathan Haidt
From The Happiness Hypothesis

May 6

"Nominate others and yourself for local, regional, and national nurse recognition awards—including AACN's Circle of Excellence program."

–Michael L. Williams, RN, MSN, CCRN

May 7

"To be seen by others as a credible, influential leader, each of us must become a healthy striver for excellence. Challenge yourself to discern whether you are driving for excellence, instead of being driven by perfectionism. I hope you will take this opportunity to pause in your day and reflect on the many roles you play in your life—and to ask: Is it excellence or is it perfectionism?"

–Denise Thornby, RN, MS

May 8

"As critical care nurses, preserving the soul means taking care that, as the inevitable craziness of even the healthiest work environment swirls around us, we stay connected to our greater purpose, our reason for being at our chosen jobs."

–Debbie Brinker, RN, MSN, CCRN, CCNS

May 9

"Knowing when to push ahead and when to quit is essential in our quest for excellence as acute and critical care nurses."

–Dave Hanson, RN, MSN, CCRN, CNS

May 10

"One lesson I learned is that the people who make a difference in our lives are not necessarily the ones who have the most credentials, the most money, or the most awards. They are simply the ones who care."

–Denise Thornby, RN, MS

May 11

"Continuous learning demands curiosity, and curiosity is the threshold to gaining insight."

–Mary Fran Tracy, RN, PhD, CCNS, CCRN, FAAN

May 12

"You are at a social event, and someone asks you what type of work you do. You reply, 'I am a nurse.' The response is: 'Oh, I could never be a nurse. I don't like blood.' Take advantage of this opportunity to share the critical thinking and crucial intervention skills that you use to save lives. Talk about the humane caring you provide and about the difference you and your actions make in the lives of your patients and their families."

—Michael L. Williams, RN, MSN, CCRN

May 13

"If our choice is to bring confident passion and positivity to our team, inspiring people to work together to improve the work environment, we will be more boldly living our purpose as critical care nurses."

—Caryl Goodyear-Bruch, RN, PhD, CCRN

May 14

"One of the things that matters most to us is our ability to deliver
top-quality critical care to our patients and their families.
Who is in a better position to address what this means
and help guide solutions than we are?"

—Connie Barden, RN, MSN, CCNS, CCRN

May 15

"If you want to grow the best tomatoes, you have to prune away
the 'suckers,' which are side shoots on the plant that compete for
nutrients with the main fruit-producing stem. Like the tomato
plant, you can also be more productive if you focus your energy.
Do you want additional expertise in nursing, critical care certification, or a graduate degree? Prune away activities that steal energy
from focusing on your goal for the best 'harvest'"!

—Cindy L. Munro, RN, ANP, PhD, FAAN

MAY 16

"The life and death situations in the ICU make you realize how easy your life is on a daily basis when you have your health."

–Heather M. Koser, RN, BSN

MAY 17

"True collaboration is an ongoing process built on mutual trust and respect."

–AACN Standards for Establishing and Sustaining
Healthy Work Environments: A Journey to Excellence

MAY 18

"You haven't failed until you quit trying."

–Anonymous

MAY 19

"New graduates or novice nurses need care, acknowledgment, and support. They need you to show them how to be highly effective critical care nurses. Although you will be challenged to give and support them as part of your team, what you will receive in return will be immeasurable."

—*Denise Thornby, RN, MS*

MAY 20

"Never underestimate what you do, for each moment presents new and meaningful ways to make a difference in the lives of others."

—*Ellen M. Harvey, MN, RN, CCRN, CNS*

May 21

"No matter how crazy things got in the ICU, we always found ways to laugh with and support one another. That made a huge difference at the end of the shift."

—Eileen Gallen Bademan, RN, BSN

May 22

"Our lives begin to end the day we come silent about things that matter."

—Martin Luther King, Jr.

May 23

"Tip: The length of tape required to secure a patient's airway will hold exactly five 4 X 6 inch photos and a rosary to the wall."

—Sonya Holder, ADN, RN, CCRN

May 24

"Compliment the newest nurses on your unit when you see them do a good job. They will be surprised and will remember your kindness."

—Denise Thornby, RN, MS

MAY 25

"The only difference between a rut and a grave…is in their dimensions."

–Ellen Glasglow

MAY 26

"You—as a critical care nurse committed to using your voice with a focus of creating change and solutions—are the one who will change the world of health care.

–Connie Barden, RN, MSN, CCRN

MAY 27

"Critical care nurses, like few other people, understand life, death, and the importance of making the most of our journey."

–Michael L. Williams, RN, MSN, CCRN

MAY 28

"Respect and value go hand in hand. When vital resources are not part of decision making, wrong decisions are bound to be made."

–Dorrie Fontaine, RN, DNSc, FAAN

MAY 29

"Tension is who you think you should be. Relaxation is who you are."

–Chinese Proverb

MAY 30

"Aside from 'Mommy,' 'Critical Care Nurse' is the moniker that I am most proud of and that has meant the most to me over time."

—Melissa A. Fitzpatrick, RN, MSN, FAAN

MAY 31

CLINICAL PEARL

A structured care conference to support the family members of an ICU patient improves communication and can reduce symptoms of posttraumatic stress disorder, anxiety, and depression in family members making end-of-life decisions.

McAdam, J.L., Puntillo, K. (2009). Symptoms Experienced by Family Members of Patients in Intensive Care Units. American Journal of Critical Care, *18(3), 200-210.*

Confidence

People with confidence have great expectations. They are accountable and committed to improving themselves. They invite feedback and communicate more often. People with confidence are collaborators. They seek other confident people as partners and develop strong bonds with them. People with confidence possess initiative to do the things that matter. They believe they can make a difference and set high expectations of success in absolutely everything they do.

Confidence is an attitude that allows us to have a positive view of ourselves that is still realistic. Confident people trust their abilities. They have a sense of control over their lives.

Confidence motivates us to act. It gives us the power to stop doing what we always did and try something new.

You might hear that annoying little voice inside you whispering "Sounds good, but don't forget, you're just a nurse." Instead of "I'm just a nurse," say "I am a good nurse; a confident nurse responsible for my patients' care." As a nurse, you represent nursing. You reflect every strength, every weakness, every good and every bad aspect of nursing. So when you transform into your confident self, you transform nursing.

Confidence is never lost. It only gets misplaced. So how do you move forward?

First, prepare yourself. What is really important to you? What have you already achieved? What do you really want to achieve?

Second, step out. Focus on the basics and set small goals that you can reasonably attain. When mistakes happen, recognize they are learning opportunities for how you can do it differently next time.

Third, accelerate your confidence. Set larger goals. Create an environment that is best for you and therefore one that is best for your patients and their families.

What a difference each one of us can make with one confident act at a time!

—Caryl Goodyear-Bruch, RN, PhD, CCRN

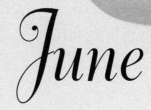

June

June 1

"Remind yourself of the meaningful work you do in critical care.
Whenever you hear yourself start the familiar refrain of 'If I were a
good nurse ...', stop! Count to 10 and savor everything
you've managed to do."

—Michael L. Williams, RN, MSN, CCRN

June 2

"Anything that gets in the way of achieving the best possible outcomes for patients must be eliminated."

—Connie Barden, RN, MSN, CCRN

June 3

"By rising above and embracing the art of possibility, new
questions are likely to reveal new opportunities."

—Dorrie Fontaine, RN, DNSc, FAAN

June 4

"There is never enough time, unless you're serving it."

—Malcolm Forbes

June 5

"Growing confidence is a reflective process, very personal
and empowering."

—Caryl Goodyear-Bruch, RN, PhD, CCRN

June 6

"As nurses caring for high acuity and critically ill patients, we live in the land of ultimate paradox, where the omnipresent reality of death casts a unique spotlight on the quality of life."

—Mary Fran Tracy, RN, PhD, CCNS, CCRN, FAAN

June 7

"I have learned that as nurses we can help provide strength with just a word, a touch, or only our presence."

—Cathy A. Yee
From A Daybook for Nurses: Making a Difference Each Day

June 8

"There are people right around you who so deserve to be recognized in even the simplest way. It's up to you to do it."

—Ellen Rudy, RN, PhD, FAAN

June 9

"Change is difficult, partly because dealing with it requires courage. I chuckle when I read the cartoon tacked to the bulletin board in my office that says, '"If change is so good ... you go first"!' The reality is that our work, our patients, our profession, and the health care system itself will continue to evolve and change. What a challenge! What an opportunity for growth."

—Denise Thornby, RN, MS

June 10

"The most precious gift we can offer others is our presence."
—Thich Nhat Hanh

June 11

"Conduct a self-inventory, a self-assessment of how safely you practice and safeguard against error."
—Denise Thornby, RN, MS

June 12

"Nothing is built on stone; all is built on sand, but we must build as if the sand were stone."
—Jorge Luis Borges

June 13

"Today, being the best means opening ourselves to the latest knowledge, stretching ourselves beyond what is familiar and secure. Being the best means listening with active self-awareness and being skilled in negotiation."

–Michael L. Williams, RN, MSN, CCRN

June 14

"It's easy for team members to isolate themselves in chaotic acute and critical care environments. But focusing on individual tasks, plans, and agendas fosters aloneness and isolates others who are there to support."

–Mary Fran Tracy, RN, PhD, CCNS, CCRN, FAAN

JUNE 15

"We are advocates. We assume their role, even if they cannot speak. We are totally responsible for their nursing care—what a truly awesome role."

—Nancy Boyd
From A Daybook for Nurses: Making a Difference Each Day

JUNE 16

"Active listening often involves silence. In some situations, there may be no words of comfort that can be given. Patients may find that a nurse's physical presence and understanding of the anguish they are experiencing are more meaningful than words of comfort."

—Marjorie Schaffer, RN, BA, MS, PhD, and
Linda Norlander, RN, BSN, MS
From Being Present: A Nurse's Resource for
End-of-Life Communication

JUNE 17

"Have you reached a point where you learn only what you need to know when you need to know it? If so, you are cutting yourself short and missing out on the exhilarating feeling that the world of learning and critical care has to offer."

–Michael L. Williams, RN, MSN, CCRN

JUNE 18

"Again and again, the impossible problem is solved when we see that the problem is only a tough decision waiting to be made."

–Robert H. Schuller

June 19

"We must be the change we wish to see in the world"
—*Mohandas K. Gandhi*

June 20

"If you chase two rabbits, you will lose them both."
—*Native American Proverb*

June 21

"To create solid, enduring improvements, we must harness the energy of the waves and use that momentum to build a strong foundation for each change we make."
—*Mary Fran Tracy, RN, PhD, CCNS, CCRN, FAAN*

JUNE 22

"I invite you to notice when fear stops you, when resignation says
you're too tired. Then notice that, instead, you can choose to
speak of the vision that inspires you with a message that
will make a difference."

—Connie Barden, RN, MSN, CCRN

JUNE 23

"Knowing when and where to disengage or engage takes courage.
It means taking a step back and looking at ourselves as
objectively as possible."

—Debbie Brinker, RN, MSN, CCRN, CCNS

June 24

"I didn't realize until I started working with critically ill patients that the strongest skills I needed were not the technical skills, but rather the ability to listen to patients and families."

—Marjorie Schaffer, RN, BA, MS, PhD, and
Linda Norlander, RN, BSN, MS
From Being Present: A Nurse's Resource for
End-of-Life Communication

June 25

"When dealing with difficult situations in critical care, know what your true message is. You must be able to clearly articulate these issues; their impact; and your request or suggestion. This will also help you explore your true motivation and avoid messaging out of anger and retribution."

—Denise Thornby, RN, MS

June 26

"Authentic leaders do not confuse enemies with opponents.
They recognize that enemies are dangerous because they seek to
harm us. Opponents keep us thinking because they look at
things in different ways."

–Kathy McCauley, RN, PhD, BC, FAAN, FAHA

June 27

"The rapidly growing approach of appreciative inquiry confirms
that identifying what we do right makes all the difference in
achieving positive outcomes."

–Caryl Goodyear-Bruch, RN, PhD, CCRN

June 28

"We must have a clear picture of the destination before we can
draw the map to get there."

–Debbie Brinker, RN, MSN, CCRN, CCNS

June 29

"It is essential to keep communication open when patients are hostile because the hostility is often not about the nurse but about the patient's fears and disappointments."

–Sharon Hudacek, RN, EdD

From Making a Difference: Stories From the Point of Care, Volume I

June 30

Clinical Pearl

Complications of overinflation of the endotracheal tube cuff include nerve palsy, tracheoesophageal fistula, tracheal wall damage, subglottic scarring or stenosis, and hoarseness.

Sole, M.L., Aragon Penoyer, D., Su, X., Jimenez, E., Kalita, S.J., Poalillo, E., et al. (2009). Assessment of Endotracheal Cuff Pressure by Continuous Monitoring: A Pilot Study. American Journal of Critical Care, *18(2), 133-143.*

It's About Time

Most of us wear watches at work. If not, there are plenty of clocks around. We're pretty skilled at keeping track of the time because so much of our work is time oriented. We administer medications at scheduled times. We measure ECG intervals by time. We predict the success of CPR based on elapsed time. We assess and reassess patients at defined moments in time.

Can you recall even one situation where you didn't feel like you needed more time? A second? A minute? An hour? A day? A week? It doesn't matter. Just a little more time. Do you ever find yourself wanting to say to time, "You're not the boss of me!" Well, it's *time* to turn the tables on time. Why not consider time based on quality instead of quantity? Instead of measuring how *much* we do, we could measure *what* we do. Instead of working harder, we could find ways to work smarter.

In changing our perspective, we would not squander time on meaningless work. Instead we would use our bold voice and boundless influence to control how we use our time, placing ourselves in the driver's seat to reclaim the priorities that only acute and critical care nurses can reclaim. For instance, we would be open to finding basic and innovative ways to keep patients safe. We would redeploy our skill in working around challenging situations toward inventing systems that work. We would expertly use the power of a positive "No" to protect and preserve nurses' valuable energy, resources, and time.

Taking control of your time and the value of quality versus quantity frees you from feeling you didn't accomplish enough. Instead, at the end of the day, your shift, or perhaps your week, you can look back at your endless To-Do list and feel satisfied with the results. Chances are your patients and their families are satisfied too.

–Dave Hanson, RN, MSN, CCRN, CNS

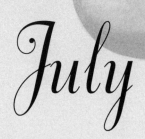

July

July 1

"The best gift a critically ill patient and his family could hope for
is a competent, vigilant, passionate and engaged critical care nurse.
Meeting the needs of those at the most vulnerable times of their
lives is an incredible privilege."

—Melissa A. Fitzpatrick, RN, MSN, FAAN

July 2

"Insights of every kind generate their own energy. By forging our
knowledge and our experience into something new, insight gener-
ates within each of us the power to grow individually as we uncover
intelligent new solutions and often, new questions."

—Mary Fran Tracy, RN, PhD, CCNS, CCRN, FAAN

July 3

"By rising above and embracing the art of possibility, new
questions are likely to reveal new opportunities."

—Dorrie Fontaine, RN, DNSc, FAAN

July 4

"Look for opportunities to share with others the kind of nursing
you do, and the rewards you feel. Use outlets such as local televi-
sion, letters to the editor in the local paper, a church bulletin,
nursing magazines, and association newsletters."

—Denise Thornby, RN, MS

July 5

"Welcome new nurses to your unit as allies. Be a role model and recognize that it is your business to help them succeed. Speak up if you believe they are not being treated fairly."

–Connie Barden, RN, MSN, CCNS, CCRN

July 6

"Enough already, I thought, as the resident gave the order for an infusion of epinephrine for a patient who had been coding off and on all evening. As a new nurse, I wasn't sure what to do, and I didn't want to 'bother' my peers, who were busy. After the patient died shortly thereafter, I regretted not calling the attending physician about the situation. That night I learned a valuable lesson about being a patient advocate."

–Cynthia Saver, RN, MS

July 7

"Most of us have been surprised, at some time or other, by
the results of our smallest efforts."

–Michael L. Williams, RN, MSN, CCRN

July 8

"Never look down on anybody unless you're helping them up."

–Jesse Jackson

July 9

"We must try to continue to hear patient voices above the
din of the machinery."

–Catherine Lopes
From A Daybook for Nurses: Making a Difference Each Day

July 10

"Our understanding of competence evolves from novice to expert.
It continually broadens and deepens to include the skills necessary
to establish and sustain healthy work environments."

–Kathy McCauley, RN, PhD, BC, FAAN, FAHA

July 11

"Get to know the families of the critically ill patients you are caring for. You will get to know the patient better through the eyes of their family. The patient will then become more of a person instead of a body you are taking care of."

–Bridget Ristagno Cabets, RN, BSN

July 12

"As critical care nurses, we must understand that our passion to care proclaims our profession as unique and elite within health care. This passion gives us our edge. But it must extend beyond patients and families to include our colleagues, especially the next generation of nurses."

—Michael L. Williams, RN, MSN, CCRN

July 13

"Using your voice doesn't require speaking in front of hundreds of people. All it requires is that you act and inform others about the essential care nurses contribute to patients."

—Connie Barden, RN, MSN, CCNS, CCRN

July 14

"It's nice to be the best, but not when being the best brings
out the worst in you."

—Rodney Dangerfield

July 15

"Nurses recognize that their dedicated efforts of caring are not only
a mark of excellence, but result in a true gift of love."

—Sharon Hudacek, RN, EdD
From A Daybook for Nurses: Making a Difference Each Day

July 16

"From success to failure is one step; from failure to
success is a long road."

—Yiddish Proverb

July 17

"Being a nurse is ultimately about the relationships we nurture with patients and their families. As nurses we want to do what is right in caring for patients. Our values are rooted in the desire (and need) to provide quality care that is dignified and respectful."

—Caryl Goodyear-Bruch, RN, PhD, CCRN

July 18

"If you are already certified, become a certification buddy and coach someone else toward achieving his or her credential."

—Dorrie Fontaine, RN, DNSc, FAAN

July 19

"Pay it forward with one coworker by doing something helpful,
something that you would not ordinarily do and something that
takes extra effort."

–Denise Thornby, RN, MS

July 20

Our greatest glory is not in never falling but in rising
every time we fall.

–Confucius

July 21

"Imagination is seeing things not as they are, but as they could be."

–Sharon M. Weinstein, MS, RN, CRNI, FAAN
From B is for Balance

July 22

"How easy it is to judge a person's behavior or appearance; how
difficult to put that aside and treat all those we meet with
gentleness and compassion."

–Elizabeth L. Santley
From A Daybook for Nurses: Making a Difference Each Day

July 23

"Sometimes rising above is as uncomplicated as shining light on a
coiled object, only to discover that it's a life-saving rope instead of
the deadly snake you imagined."

–Dorrie Fontaine, RN, DNSc, FAAN

July 24

"Twenty years from now you will be more disappointed by the
things you didn't do than by the ones you did do."

–Mark Twain

July 25

"Nurses have told me that they sometimes feel as if they're not doing enough in using their voice. Some think that a 'bold voice' has to be a 'big voice' to make a difference. We must not overlook the greater power of the messages we speak every day, wherever we practice critical care nursing."

—Connie Barden, RN, MSN, CCRN

July 26

"Every successful person needed some help to get there. For me, the real heroes are the people who remember that when they arrive. A hero turns around, looks back at where he came from, and asks what he can do to bring other people along so that they can realize their own dreams. A hero does what he can to create other leaders, never forgetting that once upon a time, he was the one with the outstretched hand."

—Earvin "Magic" Johnson

July 27

"Because the science of critical care nursing is dynamic, we are compelled to ensure that our knowledge never becomes static. We can never stop learning or we will quickly lose ground."

—Michael L. Williams, RN, MSN, CCRN

July 28

"Ignoring circumstances or behaviors that aren't in the best interest of patients, nurses, families, or others doesn't make them cease to exist. Staying quiet at best maintains circumstances as they are, leaving no room for creative and inspired solutions."

—Connie Barden, RN, MSN, CCRN

July 29

"Set aside five minutes every day to reflect on the positive impact you have had on a particular patient or family."

—Denise Thornby, RN, MS

July 30

"If you have good news and bad news, give the good first and avoid the word 'but.'"

–Cynthia Saver, RN, MS

July 31

Clinical Pearl

In a study of nurses' perceptions about allowing family members to be present during resuscitation, the authors reported that nurses with greater self-confidence offered resuscitation presence more often and nurses who were certified invited family presence more often than did noncertified nurses.

Twibell, R.S., Siela, D., Riwitis, C., Wheatley, J., Riegle, T., Bousman, D., et al.
Nurses perception about the benefits of family presence during resuscitation. (2008). American Journal of Critical Care, *17(2), 101-111.*

Leaders—What About Them?

Authenticity literally means to conform to fact, making the authentic person worthy of trust, reliance, or belief. An authentic leader genuinely understands what happens at the point of care and successfully translates his or her vision so it becomes relevant at the frontline. Nurse leaders play a key role in retaining staff by shaping the health care practice environment to produce quality outcomes for their staff and patients.

A wise leader knows that a poorly translated vision left in the hands of an uncommitted team means nothing more than idle dreaming. Transformational leadership is the essential precursor to patient safety, successful organizational change, and an organization's competitive position. Transformational leadership involves influencing the choices that individuals and groups make in order to achieve lasting and positive change.

Leaders are obligated to translate their vision so everyone in the organization can understand his or her part in achieving it. But don't wait until you hear from your leader. Be proactive. Schedule time with each of your nurse leaders—CNO, director, manager, advanced practice nurse—to inquire about their vision. When you take time to learn more about them and their vision, you will most likely discover you share more similarities than differences.

In the leadership classic, *Flight of the Buffalo*, James Belasco and Ralph Stayer refer to the "eternal circle" of doing, learning, and changing. Mistakes and fear are consistently two of the most effective teachers. Fearful leaders teach us what happens when we allow ourselves to become paralyzed. Leaders who make mistakes teach us how to move beyond fear. Have you known leaders skilled in overcoming adversity? Have you worked with leaders who truly viewed failure as their friend and not an enemy to be avoided?

If only I could be like _____. You fill in the blank.

—Dave Hanson, RN, MSN, CCRN, CNS

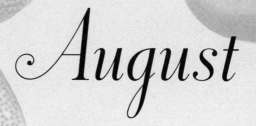

August

AUGUST 1

"A lived contribution becomes possible when we commit to work together, moving forward in our personal competence journeys, relying on and celebrating the contributions of our equally committed colleagues."

–Kathy McCauley, RN, PhD, BC, FAAN, FAHA

AUGUST 2

"I've sought to master a practical way to approach difficult situations—one that spells the acronym AIR2 and prompts me to be: Attentive, Intelligent, Reasonable, and Responsive."

–Dorrie Fontaine, RN, DNSc, FAAN

August 3

"Outstanding solutions invent new ways to handle a challenge. They blend the best of the evidence with the wisdom of experience."

—Connie Barden, RN, MSN, CCRN

August 4

"Do not go where the path may lead, go instead where there is no path and leave a trail."

—Ralph Waldo Emerson

August 5

"I don't see anything unusual about a man being a critical care nurse, do you?"

—Michael L. Williams, RN, MSN, CCRN

August 6

"Reach out to an inexperienced physician to help him or her understand how to better care for critically ill patients, talk with families, be a good team member to other nurses and help them gain an understanding of nursing's contributions."

–Denise Thornby, RN, MS

August 7

"As critical care nurses, we treasure the privilege of caring and keep the sacred space between our patients and us close to our hearts. Keeping this in focus will keep us safe and whole on our journey."

–Michael L. Williams, RN, MSN, CCRN

August 8

"Remember that 'no' can be a complete sentence. This means that it's perfectly acceptable to say 'no' without any further explanation."

–Sharon M. Weinstein, MS, RN, CRNI, FAAN
From B is for Balance

August 9

"I may not be able to fix the problems of the world, but I can use the art of nursing to help heal the body and the heart."

–Angie Riches
From A Daybook for Nurses: Making a Difference Each Day

AUGUST 10

"Nurse leaders must fully embrace the imperative of a healthy
work environment, authentically live it, and engage
others in its achievement."

—AACN Standards for Establishing and Sustaining
Healthy Work Environments: A Journey to Excellence

AUGUST 11

"Repeated studies confirm that the leadership approach at the top
sets the tone for true collaboration and effective decision-making;
everyone is empowered to optimize their contribution."

—*Debbie Brinker, RN, MSN, CCRN, CCNS*

August 12

"When you make a mistake, don't beat yourself up. Instead, think about what you would do differently next time and move on."

–Cynthia Saver, RN, MS

August 13

"Skilled communication protects and advances collaborative relationships."

–AACN Standards for Establishing and Sustaining Healthy Work Environments: A Journey to Excellence

August 14

"As we shape our journeys, they also shape us. Whether this journey is professional or personal, it is essential that we keep moving."

–Michael L. Williams, RN, MSN, CCRN

AUGUST 15

"The ICU is stressful and good nurses know what to do and execute their skills under huge amounts of pressure. Good ICU nurses master this skill and then everyday decisions are easier to make."

–Heather M. Koser, RN, BSN

AUGUST 16

"Dwelling on fault and blame will mire a conversation. Focusing on solutions gives the interaction a goal and a purpose."

–Connie Barden, RN, MSN, CCNS, CCRN

AUGUST 17

"Never has it been more important for all health care professionals to work together. 'United we stand; divided we fall' pretty much sums up the situation."

–Denise Thornby, RN, MS

August 18

"I have always felt that in order to be successful and have a long career in critical care nursing that you should have an outside hobby—an activity that not only balances the stress of your work, but replenishes your battery. I believe in working hard and playing harder."

—Victoria A. Kark, RN, CCNS, CCRN, MSN

August 19

"Authentic leaders recognize the amusement in their experience and use it to establish and sustain healthy work environments where everyone is inspired to connect with their purpose and make a lived contribution."

—Kathy McCauley, RN, PhD, BC, FAAN, FAHA

AUGUST 20

"One trait that many critical care nurses struggle with is perfectionism. As my family and friends are quick to point out, it is also a tendency of mine. However, I have come to realize that perfectionism is not a healthy pursuit of excellence."

–Denise Thornby, RN, MS

AUGUST 21

"Being driven by our purpose—to provide the best outcomes for a patient—becomes the vehicle to create the solutions even in difficult circumstances."

–Connie Barden, RN, MSN, CCRN

August 22

"With purpose comes all kinds of possibilities for taking confident
actions that matter to our patients."

–Caryl Goodyear-Bruch, RN, PhD, CCRN

August 23

"In our work as nurses, we have tremendous power to influence the
outcomes of our patients, to put their care first, above all else."

–Dave Hanson, RN, MSN, CCRN, CNS

August 24

"Courage is the power to let go of the familiar."

–Raymond Lindquist

August 25

"Let's commit to creating work environments where caring for each other isn't the exception, but expected and valued."

—Michael L. Williams, RN, MSN, CCRN

August 26

"Let us, as nurses, never forget the purpose of our work is to care for patients, no matter the circumstances that brought them to us."

—Sharon Hudacek, RN, EdD
From Making a Difference: Stories From the Point of Care, Volume II

August 27

"The next time we are faced with an impossible situation, where a positive outcome seems far from reality, just sit back and *believe*."

—Maryann Godshall
From A Daybook for Nurses: Making A Difference Each Day

August 28

"'I'm dying!' I'll never forget when a patient (who had just been shifted to do not resuscitate status) sat straight up in his CCU bed and said those words. The patient's nurse gave him some sedation, but, most importantly, calmed him by touching him and leaning in closer to show him she was there for him."

–Cynthia Saver, RN, MS

August 29

"A study of 19,000 certified nurses in the U.S. and Canada found that certified nurses overwhelmingly reported that certification enabled them to experience personal growth and feel more satisfied in their work."

–Connie Barden, RN, MSN, CCNS, CCRN

August 30

"If we are to improve the health of our work environments and provide quality, patient-centered care, we must have competent teams who value and demonstrate true collaboration."

—Caryl Goodyear-Bruch, RN, PhD, CCRN

August 31

Clinical Pearl

Early mobility in critically ill patients is not only feasible and safe, but has the potential to prevent or treat complications of critical illness.

Perme, C., Chandrashekar, R. Early Mobility and Walking Program for Patients in Intensive Care Units: Creating a Standard of Care. (2009). American Journal of Critical Care, 18(3), 212-221.

MENTORING NEW NURSES

The work and the workload we must manage to be able to care for all the patients in our ICUs and acute care areas are intense. The facts that patients are sicker than ever, that technology has increased, that support services are scarcer, that medical interventions are more complicated, and that there is a shortage of nursing staff can be overwhelming. And yet, we must provide a supportive, nurturing environment that can foster the growth and development of new staff. We must bring novice nurses into our units and provide them with adequate support to become fully competent acute and critical care nurses. Each new hire into our units is a gift and should be treated as such. They should be greeted with open arms of encouragement. We have a professional obligation to coach, mentor, and pass on our expertise to others.

Some tips to help you help our novice nurses:

- Respond openly and honestly to their questions.
  This provides
  them with an excellent learning opportunity and helps them feel comfortable when other matters of uncertainty arise.
- Encourage them to take care of themselves
- Help them realize they are learning and gaining skills.
- Tell stories of experiences you had as a new nurse (we all have them!).
- Give them articles or suggest books to read.
- Encourage them to accept more challenging patients.
- Relieve them when they need help.

New graduates or novice nurses need care, acknowledgment, and support. They need you to show them how to be highly effective acute and critical care nurses. Although you will be challenged to give and support these new "gifts" to your team, what you will receive in return will be immeasurable.

–Denise Thornby, RN, MS

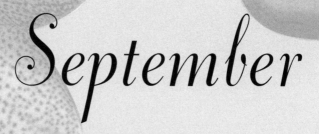

September

SEPTEMBER 1

"Hope is like a bird that senses the dawn and carefully starts to
sing while it is still dark."

—Anonymous

SEPTEMBER 2

"A little touch and a few soft words make a difference to the
patient and their families."

—Susanne Thees, RN

SEPTEMBER 3

"Our contributions to critical care will nurture our souls and
define new realities of practice in our units."

—Kathy McCauley, RN, PhD, BC, FAAN, FAHA

September 4

"The moment we begin to fear the opinions of others and hesitate to tell the truth that is in us, and from motives of policy are silent when we should speak, the divine floods of light and life no longer flow into our soul."

–Elizabeth Cady Stanton

September 5

"Teamwork has become more important than ever to success in critical care in today's health care world. Benjamin Franklin was not far off when he said, 'If we don't hang together, we will surely hang separately.'"

–Michael L. Williams, RN, MSN, CCRN

SEPTEMBER 6

"You can't do anything about the length of your life, but you can
do something about its width and depth."

—Shira Tehrani

SEPTEMBER 7

"Exercising our choices empowers us. When you are frightened or
uncertain about a new procedure or patient population, make the
choice to gain the knowledge or seek the mentoring you need to
become more competent and confident."

—Denise Thornby, RN, MS

SEPTEMBER 8

"Several studies confirm nurses' critical surveillance role. We are
the eyes, ears, and hands of the health system every minute of
every day."

—Kathy McCauley, RN, PhD, BC, FAAN, FAHA

September 9

"Our deepest fear is not that we are inadequate. Our deepest fear is that we are powerful beyond measure. It is our light, not our darkness that frightens us most. We ask ourselves, 'Who am I to be brilliant, gorgeous, talented, and famous?' Actually, who are you not to be? You are a child of God. Your playing small does not serve the world. ...When we let our own light shine, we unconsciously give other people permission to do the same. As we are liberated from our own fear, our presence automatically liberates others."

—Nelson Mandela

September 10

"Every nurse wants competence, quality, and an environment that supports nursing excellence. So does every employer. Every patient and family certainly needs it. And, we all have a role to play."

—Connie Barden, RN, MSN, CCNS, CCRN

September 11

"Leadership driven by love and caring means units where meeting the needs of patients and families is the focus—units where the precious resource of nurses is respected, valued, and trusted."

—Dorrie Fontaine, RN, DNSc, FAAN

September 12

"Being there to make a contribution means making a commitment to use your best talents, to stay engaged, to intentionally make a difference. It means truly living your contribution."

—Kathy McCauley, RN, PhD, BC, FAAN, FAHA

September 13

"We all know that uncertainty and critical care do not mix willingly. One of our most endearing qualities as critical care nurses is our inherent need to always be certain—our need to be the very best."

–Michael L. Williams, RN, MSN, CCRN

September 14

"One isn't necessarily born with courage, but one is born with potential. Without courage, we cannot practice any other virtue with consistency. We can't be kind, true, merciful, generous, or honest."

–Maya Angelou

SEPTEMBER 15

"Thoughtfully transform facts into knowledge. Ask good questions
and expect good answers."

—Dorrie Fontaine, RN, DNSc, FAAN

SEPTEMBER 16

"Skilled listeners are generous listeners. Generous listening means
allowing others to have their point of view and being determined
to find what is 'good' in it."

—Connie Barden, RN, MSN, CCRN

September 17

"The word courage is derived from the French word *coeur*, which
means heart. Thus, practicing courage means exercising
acts of the heart."

–Denise Thornby, RN, MS

September 18

"The work will always be there when you get back from break
or lunch, but at least you will feel better."

–Susan Gerhardt, MSN, RN

September 19

"The only job where you start at the top is digging a hole."
—Anonymous

September 20

"When you get to the end of your rope, tie a knot and hang on."
—Franklin D. Roosevelt

September 21

"There are two important bridges that take us from looking inward to reaching out. Change is the first; the other is discovery."
—Michael L. Williams, RN, MSN, CCRN

SEPTEMBER 22

"Courage, faith, strength, and love—nurses report that these
and many more attributes are the gifts they get from patients
and their families."

–Sharon Hudacek, RN, EdD
From Making a Difference: Stories From the Point of Care, Volume II

SEPTEMBER 23

"Learn how to focus your energy on the priority of each present
moment rather than squandering it disjointedly among a jumble
of competing priorities."

–Dave Hanson, RN, MSN, CCRN, CNS

September 24

"The ability to simplify means to eliminate the unnecessary so
that the necessary may speak."

–Hans Hofmann

September 25

"When we fail to identify and acknowledge reality, we delude
ourselves and make overcoming issues that undermine our
dream-driven intentions difficult, if not impossible."

–Denise Thornby, RN, MS

September 26

"I am convinced that listening is so important that unless we become focused and committed listeners, nothing will change."

—Connie Barden, RN, MSN, CCRN

September 27

"Even in difficult times, there still are great reasons to be a nurse."

—Anonymous

September 28

"It takes two to quarrel, but only one to end it."
—Spanish Proverb

September 29

"Self-knowledge helps me to become empowered and to empower others. It reaffirms that I make a difference because I am here today."
—Kathy McCauley, RN, PhD, BC, FAAN, FAHA

SEPTEMBER 30

CLINICAL PEARL

Heart murmurs are commonly found in children and infants
and do not always indicate heart disease.

–Patricia Vanderpool, MSN, APN-BC, ANPE

Moral Distress

Your patient lies comatose in his ICU bed, his ventilator humming, ECG beeping along, and tubes hanging out of nearly every orifice. Your gut instinct tells you it's time for a do not resuscitate (DNR) order; the doctors agree, but the patient's family doesn't—firmly believing the patient's reflexive hand grasp means he will wake up soon. As the days drag on, you weary of the situation and find yourself sad and irritable.

Situations like this create moral distress in critical care and acute care nurses. Moral distress occurs when your personal values and ethical obligations are in conflict with what is happening around you. Nurses are at risk for moral distress. We spend the most time with the patient, giving the drugs, hanging the IV bags, and helping with the chest tube insertion and other procedures that may have little chance of changing the ultimate outcome.

Unfortunately, too many of us suffer in silence, unable to put a name to our problem, not realizing it's the source of our negative emotion. The American Association of Critical-Care Nurses developed a model to help nurses work through moral distress. It's called *The 4A's to Rise Above Moral Distress*:

Ask: Determine if moral distress is present.

Affirm: Validate your perceptions with others and make a commitment to address the issue.

Assess: Identify the sources of the distress and decide if you are ready to act.

Act: Plan to take action and implement strategies needed to make change.

Open communication is the prescription for prevention, as well as the antidote for, moral distress. Don't hesitate to call a multidisciplinary team meeting (including nurses, doctors, social workers, clergy, and other key personnel) to discuss a situation causing your distress. Remember, other members of the team may be suffering in silence from the same distress and welcome the opportunity to talk about it.

–*Cynthia Saver, RN, MS*

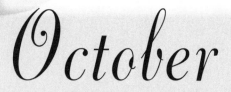

October

OCTOBER 1

"The best and most beautiful things in this world cannot be seen or
even heard, but must be felt with the heart."

–Helen Keller

OCTOBER 2

"Role modeling for men in nursing is a challenge, because each of
us is unique in his own right. Nevertheless, I am convinced that
bringing male and female perspectives equally to the point of care
will enrich our profession and benefit our patients and
their families."

–Michael L. Williams, RN, MSN, CCRN

133

OCTOBER 3

"Reframing what failure means may mean reframing what
success means."

—Caryl Goodyear-Bruch, RN, PhD, CCRN

OCTOBER 4

"If the going is really easy, beware; you may be headed downhill."

—Anonymous

OCTOBER 5

"Two rules of thumb to practice by: If it doesn't feel right,
it probably isn't; if you wouldn't do it to your mom, don't do
it to your patient."

—Charles Reed, MSN, RN, CNRN

October 6

"Hearing that we are not perfect may be difficult for critical care nurses. Yet, learning from criticism can help us keep our dreams on track and make the changes needed. Instead of viewing circumstances as we would like them to be, we should listen and learn from others' thoughts, insights, criticisms, and challenges."

—Denise Thornby, RN, MS

October 7

"Vulnerability and the need for support are not functions of chronological or developmental age. The healing value of a person's family persists throughout life. Ask any nurse whose family member has been hospitalized. The view is different from the other side of the care equation."

—Mary Fran Tracy, RN, PhD, CCNS, CCRN, FAAN

OCTOBER 8

"Courage enables us to see the landscape as it is, to consider possibility, and to respond with generosity. It reminds us that nursing is the most optimistic of sciences, because human caring makes a difference, makes everything possible."

–Dorrie Fontaine, RN, DNSc, FAAN

OCTOBER 9

"If competence is not optional, then incompetence cannot be ignored. In fact, we are ethically obligated, not only to maintain our own competence, but also to support one another in becoming competent and to call out incompetence when it appears."

–Kathy McCauley, RN, PhD, BC, FAAN, FAHA

OCTOBER 10

"Actively listen to other people's perspectives and find the lesson in
their message. Remember to seek first to understand and
then be understood."

—Michael L. Williams, RN, MSN, CCRN

OCTOBER 11

"To be truly effective critical care nurses need to create workplaces
that support our optimal contribution to care that is driven by the
needs of patients and their families, and we must be able to speak
the truth in such a way that it is heard and acted upon."

—Denise Thornby, RN, MS

October 12

"A bold voice is a committed voice. It will be heard in everyday interactions—at the bedside, in the nurses' station, during staff and faculty meetings, and among peers—where the standard of excellence we demand for our patients and ourselves is reflected."

–Connie Barden, RN, MSN, CCRN

October 13

"Dissatisfaction alone is usually not enough to bring about change. We also need a vision of how things can be better and people must believe that the vision is realistic and will work."

–Debbie Brinker, RN, MSN, CCRN, CCNS

October 14

"Why not go out on a limb? Isn't that where the fruit is?"
—Frank Scully

October 15

"Experienced nurses actively mentoring new nurses offer a lived contribution. Thinking aloud as they assess a patient shares their wisdom about a complex patient."
—Kathy McCauley, RN, PhD, BC, FAAN, FAHA

October 16

"If you don't learn from your mistakes, there's no sense making them."
—Anonymous

OCTOBER 17

"Learning to handle 'crucial conversations' when the stakes are high will bring the positive results we need in dealing with patient safety, moral distress, and collaboration—three critical issues that spill over into every corner of our work."

–Dorrie Fontaine, RN, DNSc, FAAN

OCTOBER 18

"Highlight the great work that your fellow nurses do. Become a regular user of your hospital's employee recognition program to recognize their efforts."

–Michael L. Williams, RN, MSN, CCRN

OCTOBER 19

"Take the first step in faith. You don't have to see the whole staircase, just take the first step."

—Martin Luther King, Jr.

OCTOBER 20

"Change is central to practice, and it is particularly characteristic of critical care practice. Practice today is different from yesterday, and it will be different tomorrow. We should welcome change when that change is in a direction that honors our hopes for patients."

—Cindy L. Munro, RN, PhD, ANP
From American Journal of Critical Care, *2009, Vol. 18, pp. 188-190*

October 21

"When we engage and open ourselves to others, we create strength of partnership, which enables us to achieve goals that are not possible alone."

—Denise Thornby, RN, MS

October 22

"It is no surprise that nurses might wonder how they, as individuals, can make a difference in this madness we call health care. Yet, no one else is more qualified, more called, more prepared, and more driven to make the changes needed to create a better future for health care."

—Connie Barden, RN, MSN, CCRN

October 23

"We as nurses are the creators and sharers of insights that ensure our patients' wishes are honored—that they are not in pain and that they are better for the care we provide."

—Mary Fran Tracy, RN, PhD, CCNS, CCRN, FAAN

October 24

"Nurses must be recognized and must recognize others for the value each brings to the work of the organization."

–AACN Standards for Establishing and Sustaining
Healthy Work Environments: A Journey to Excellence

OCTOBER 25

"Life must be understood backwards ... but it must be lived forwards."

—Søren Kierkegaard

OCTOBER 26

"Sometimes the most important thing in a whole day is the rest we take between two deep breaths."

—Etty Hillesum
From B is for Balance

OCTOBER 27

"Compliment other critical care nurses in public. Proudly brag to their colleagues and other team members about the wonderful job they do."

—Michael L. Williams, RN, MSN, CCRN

OCTOBER 28

"To be a fully expert critical care nurse, you must not only have expert technical skills, knowledge, and judgment, but also effective people skills. The truth is that those who possess a high degree of emotional intelligence are the ones who truly become star performers within their profession."

—Denise Thornby, RN, MS

OCTOBER 29

"Challenges are what make life interesting; overcoming them is what makes life meaningful."

—Joshua J. Marine

October 30

"What is a 'bold' voice? It isn't a blaming voice or a whining voice.
It doesn't argue about who is right or wrong or about whose
fault it is that we are faced with challenges. A bold voice
moves past complaints to look for solutions."

–Connie Barden, RN, MSN, CCRN

October 31

Clinical Pearl

"Prendergast and colleagues evaluated the oral health status of intubated patients in a neuroscience intensive care unit and described
the effect of oral care on intracranial pressure (ICP). They found
oral care was associated with no adverse effects in patients whose
ICP was less than 20 mm Hg before oral care was instituted. Also,
in patients whose ICP was higher than 20 mm Hg before oral care,
ICP decreased 76% or remained stable during and after oral care."

Prendergast, V., Hallberg, I.R., Jahnke, H., Kleiman, C., Hagell, P.
(2009). Oral Health, Ventilator-Associated Pneumonia, and Intracrani-
al Pressure in Intubated Patients in a Neuroscience Intensive Care Unit.
American Journal of Critical Care, *18(4), 368-376.*

Gratitude, Hope, Confidence, and Acorns

Thanksgiving—the time of the year when many of us reflect on what we have and for what we are grateful. Our families, our friends, yes, even our jobs! But have you ever wondered why gratitude generally happens after the fact? What if it became an ongoing part of our journey instead of a destination?

If we hadn't withheld gratitude until something happened, we might have started the hurricane season by thanking the talented and caring health professionals who would care for the hurricane victims. Or, we would have appreciated our financial gifts, however modest, while we enjoyed them before a down economy took some of them away.

Gratitude focuses us in good times and bad. Whether our gratitude is low-key or exuberant, it renews our sense of hope. Hope, after all, is our stock-in-trade as nurses, isn't it? Our patients and their families count on us to bring them hope. Hope that pain will be eased. Hope for a cure. Hope for a peaceful death. Hope that they will never be alone.

Hope, in turn, bolsters our confidence. Confidence that we can return the love and caring of our family and friends. Confidence that, without the gifts we bring to ourselves and those around us, the world would be a very dreary place.

The acorns? Oak trees and acorns are ancient symbols. Some people describe acorns as symbolizing the potential for great power in a small but potent package. Or, as botanists joke, even the greatest oak was once a little nut. For many, acorns represent endurance, strength, and hope for the future.

Thank you for the extraordinary gifts you bring to nursing and the hopeful confidence with which you share them.

–Caryl Goodyear-Bruch, RN, PhD, CCRN

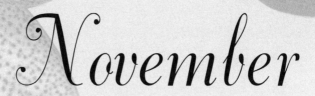

November

November 1

"The secret to happiness is not in doing what one likes to do, but
in liking what one has to do."

—Anonymous

November 2

"Collaboration is not necessarily about agreeing. However, it is
about respecting the contributions and perspectives of others who
are members of the interdisciplinary team."

—Denise Thornby, RN, MS

November 3

"I believe we share three non-negotiable core values in our professional life as acute and critical care nurses: Patients and families are our first core value, safety is the second, and reliability is the third."

–Dave Hanson, RN, MSN, CCRN, CNS

November 4

"As critical care nurses, we often display some endearing traits. For example:

- We are high-achievers who border on perfectionism.
- We blithely take on responsibilities that seem beyond belief to mere mortals.
- We buy into the thinking that good isn't enough, that better will be just around the bend."

–Michael L. Williams, RN, MSN, CCRN

November 5

"We are blessed with competent, compassionate, and committed nurses, though too few to meet the need. But that means the value of each contribution is ever more precious, and it becomes ever more important that it be lived."

–*Kathy McCauley, RN, PhD, BC, FAAN, FAHA*

November 6

"When you're having conflict with someone, take time to remember that every person has a story—and it's not always a happy one. Think about *why* a person might be acting the way he or she is and listen even harder."

–*Cynthia Saver, RN, MS*

November 7

"We are like tea bags—we don't know our own strength until we're in hot water."

—Sister Busche

November 8

"Fear is a powerful barrier to overcome. However, the risks of remaining silent far outweigh the risks of speaking up."

—Denise Thornby, RN, MS

November 9

"Care with knowledge and confidence, and you will gain the trust of your patient and their loved ones."

—Susanne Thees, RN

November 10

"There are challenges and rewards when you think of a bold and powerful voice as representing your commitment to a new way of being. The challenge is that speaking with a bold and powerful voice isn't a one-time event. When you are genuinely committed to having your voice matter, it never ends."

—Connie Barden, RN, MSN, CCRN

November 11

"In this life we cannot do great things. We can only do small things with great love."

—Mother Theresa

November 12

"Give credit. Say thank you…What should we take credit for as nurses and, as a result, stand taller?"

–Dorrie Fontaine, RN, DNSc, FAAN

November 13

"Excellence isn't an endpoint. It's a lifelong commitment to pursue relentlessly."

–Debbie Brinker, RN, MSN, CCRN, CCNS

November 14

"Make time to write a 'formal' letter acknowledging another
nurse's truly outstanding work. Remember to send a
copy to his or her boss."

–Michael L. Williams, RN, MSN, CCRN

November 15

"The unique contributions we live as nurses have never been more
explicit, with science, the best available evidence, and exquisite
clinical judgment as our guides."

–Kathy McCauley, RN, PhD, BC, FAAN, FAHA

November 16

"We have the best sick-care in the world. The problem is we don't
have good health care."

—Jocelyn Elders, MD
From A Daybook for Nurse Leaders and Mentors

November 17

"Some simple rules to help navigate the chaotic waves that are present in critical care today: Show up. Be present. Tell the truth. Keep
the vision as your beacon. And, make waves!"

—Denise Thornby, RN, MS

November 18

"Life is like the carpool lane. The only way to get to your
destination quickly is to take some people with you."

—Peter Ward

November 19

"One hundred percent of the shots you don't take don't go in."

—Wayne Gretzky

November 20

"Critical care nurses have a proud legacy of leadership and influence. We can be counted on to step up to challenges to ensure
that we provide the best care for our patients."

—Denise Thornby, RN, MS

November 21

"Speak purposefully and enthusiastically about what it takes to be an expert critical care nurse. Caring is vital, but without expert knowledge, skill, judgment, and decision making, it doesn't save lives."

—Connie Barden, RN, MSN, CCNS, CCRN

November 22

"Terminating care is always difficult, even when it's the wish of the patient or the family. But it takes a particular perspective to realize that the act of termination is caring at its most fundamental level."

—Sharon Hudacek, RN, EdD
From Making a Difference: Stories From the Point of Care, Volume I

November 23

"Asking questions is foundational in finding enduring solutions to
improve our patients' quality of care."

—Mary Fran Tracy, RN, PhD, CCNS, CCRN, FAAN

November 24

"Talents are our natural abilities that, when used, generate energy
and are intrinsically rewarding to us."

—Nancy Dickenson-Hazard, RN, MSN, FAAN
From Ready, Set, Go Lead!

November 25

"Confident people understand one basic rule: control your attitude instead of letting attitudes control you."

–Caryl Goodyear-Bruch, RN, PhD, CCRN

November 26

"We need to be aware of our vulnerability as well as consider the vulnerability of our co-workers in managing conflict. Sometimes we have the strength to support others, and sometimes we are the ones who need support."

–Marjorie Schaffer, RN, BA, MS, PhD, and
Linda Norlander, RN, BSN, MS
From Being Present: A Nurse's Resource for
End-of-Life Communication

November 27

"The road to success is lined with many tempting parking spaces."
—Traditional Proverb

November 28

"It has been said that courage is not the absence of fear. It is the willingness to take action even in the presence of fear."
—Connie Barden, RN, MSN, CCRN

November 29

"The debate over health care is not complete until critical care nurses are heard."
—Denise Thornby, RN, MS

November 30

Clinical Pearl

The systemic inflammatory response syndrome (SIRS) is a severe hyperinflammatory condition frequently observed in critically ill patients. NeSmith and colleagues show that the SIRS scores on ICU admission predicted ICU length of stay. The SIRS score is based on the SIRS criteria, where one point is assigned to each of four criteria:

1. A temperature of less than 36°C or greater than 38°C

2. A heart rate higher than 90/min

3. A respiratory rate higher than 20/min or $PaCO_2$ less than 32 mm Hg

4. A white blood cell count greater than 12,000/µL, less than 4,000/µL, or a presence of 10% immature neutrophils.

   - This score predicts deadly complications seen in the ICU, including infection and sepsis.

   - The SIRS score is a quick and easy-to-use bedside tool.

   - The SIRS score may be useful when planning preventive care, including a targeted time frame for patient and family education, reducing skin breakdown, and planning for discharge needs.

NeSmith, E.G., Weinrich, S.P., Andrews, J.O., Medeiros, R.S., Hawkins, M.L., Weinrich, M. (2009). Systemic Inflammatory Response Syndrome Score and Race As Predictors of Length of Stay in the Intensive Care Unit. American Journal of Critical Care, *18(4), 339-347.*

Taking Care of Ourselves—Renewing

The holiday season has become relentlessly fast-paced. Our daily lives may be so hectic that we find ourselves struggling to engage in their renewing opportunity.

After all, critically ill patients don't take holidays. Nor do their families. Add the sometimes burdensome activities of the season—shopping, family commitment, social obligations, or perhaps individual loneliness and isolation—and we might wonder how we can also make time for renewal.

But how can we not? How can we care for others when we are drained of energy? Perhaps the challenge lies in sorting out what renewal means to each of us. Renewal is about perspective. Make it a chore and our burden increases. Make it a gift and our load is transformed.

Knitting. Needlepoint. Photography. Sleeping for nine hours. Reading. Hiking. Dancing. Singing, even off key. Savoring freshly baked bread or the health-promoting qualities of dark chocolate. Jogging. Power walking. Delighting in the moon as it sparkles on the water or a fresh blanket of winter snow. I hope you find yourself subconsciously adding to the list.

Above all, renewal is about caring for yourself. Celebrating yourself in meaningful ways that leave you refreshed and mindful of everything that makes a difference in your life.

Such magic at only the price of our attention! No need to grasp greedily at such moments: They come upon us naturally—yes, repeatedly—in the utter simplicity and fullness of life. There is more than enough for us all.

Care for yourself so you'll have the energy, renewed passion, and commitment to optimally care for your patients and their families. Celebrate your relationships and accomplishments as an individual and as a team. Renew your passion for the difficult, rewarding work you do and recommit to engage and transform your personal practice and your work environment. Maybe you will find yourself renewed and celebrating that you are truly an extraordinary nurse.

–Debbie Brinker, RN, MSN, CCRN, CCNS

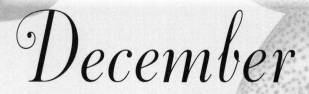

December

December 1

"Ask your patients or their families at the start of each shift what they'd like to make happen that day. Every time you can help make something happen, you'll feel great."

–Michael L. Williams, RN, MSN, CCRN

December 2

"Confidence isn't accidental. It's intentional."

–Caryl Goodyear-Bruch, RN, PhD, CCRN

December 3

"A leader has to be sensitive to the people who are creative, to the people who are competitive, to the people who are into control, and to the people who are into collaboration."

–Daniel J. Pesut, APRN, BC, PhD, FAAN
From A Daybook for Nurse Leaders and Mentors

December 4

"We practice nursing through relationships. If we are to be effective critical care nurses, we must always be able to have effective relationships with our patients, their families and our coworkers, as well as everyone else in our work setting."

–Denise Thornby, RN, MS

DECEMBER 5

"What we see depends mainly on what we look for."
–Sir John Lubbock

DECEMBER 6

"Nurses must be relentless in pursuing and fostering true
collaboration."

–AACN Standards for Establishing and Sustaining
Healthy Work Environments: A Journey to Excellence

DECEMBER 7

"Success usually comes to those who are too busy to be
looking for it."
–Henry David Thoreau

December 8

"We must listen to the bold voices that deliver the difficult messages. We do not need to wait for higher authorities to do what needs to be done. Nurses are the highest authority when it comes to addressing pain and creating safe and humane environments."

—Connie Barden, RN, MSN, CCRN

December 9

"Make time for a personal debriefing at the end of every work shift. Highlight what you accomplished by creating a 'done' list instead of a 'to-do' list."

—Michael L. Williams, RN, MSN, CCRN

December 10

"So much has been given to me, I have not time to ponder over that which has been denied."

—Helen Keller

December 11

"Despite my best efforts, when a persistent and complex challenge doesn't change, I learned that this is a signal—a signal for me to overcome well-conditioned reflexes and consider the challenge from another angle."

—Dorrie Fontaine, RN, DNSc, FAAN

December 12

"Make failure your teacher, not your undertaker."
–Zig Ziglar

December 13

"Embrace physicians and other team members as equal colleagues.
Clearly state your suggestions about the patient's care, and listen
carefully to theirs."
–Connie Barden, RN, MSN, CCNS, CCRN

December 14

"It is not suffering as such that is most deeply feared but suffering
that degrades."
–Susan Sontag

December 15

"Have you made certain that you have the skills, abilities, competencies, and experiences needed to care for any patient presented to you?"

–Denise Thornby, RN, MS

December 16

"You can never be happy at the expense of the happiness of others."

–Chinese Proverb

December 17

"Don't follow your dreams; chase them."

—Unknown

December 18

"Remember 'quiet time' from your childhood? Bring it back each day, even if it's only for a few minutes."

Cynthia Saver, RN, MS

December 19

"In effective high-energy teams, everyone knows their roles and can be relied on to deliver on their accountabilities."

—Caryl Goodyear-Bruch, RN, PhD, CCRN

December 20

"Do you report errors or 'near-misses' and examine the opportunities to prevent those errors in the future?"

—Denise Thornby, RN, MS

December 21

"Keep focused on patients and their families. When access to care and quality are compromised, every patient suffers. Some die. A scarcity of nurses means less access and quality of health care for the public. And for you."

—Michael L. Williams, RN, MSN, CCRN

DECEMBER 22

"Learning to act under life and death pressure is an acquired skill, that, when mastered, enlightens one to the ease and pleasures of everyday life."

–Heather M. Koser, RN, BSN

DECEMBER 23

"Clinical nurses can improve relationships with physicians and quality of patient care by participating in interdisciplinary collaborative patient rounds, resolving conflict constructively, performing competently, and demonstrating self-confidence."

–Claudia Schmalenberg, RN, MSN, and Marlene Kramer, RN, PhD
From "Nurse-Physician Relationships in Hospitals:
20,000 Nurses Tell Their Story" (Critical Care Nurse, *Vol.29/No.1; pp*
74-83)

DECEMBER 24

"The only way to have a friend is to be one."
–Ralph Waldo Emerson

DECEMBER 25

"We are not human beings on a spiritual journey. We are spiritual beings on a human journey"
–Stephen Covey

DECEMBER 26

"By simply shifting to a perspective of openness and possibility—by rising above, so to speak—we can transform with hope some of the thorniest challenges we face."
–Dorrie Fontaine, RN, DNSc, FAAN

December 27

"To have very effective teams within our critical care units,
we must confront those who show a lack of interpersonal
effectiveness.'"

–Denise Thornby, RN, MS

December 28

"Just as we need to nourish our bodies, we need to nourish our
minds and our skills. When you have to skip lunch, you eventually
eat later. If you don't have time to read that article or attend that
educational program now, make time to do so later."

–Michael L. Williams, RN, MSN, CCRN

DECEMBER 29

"Our work relies on relationships—establishing, sustaining, and building them...Aren't relationships at the heart of everything we do?"

Caryl Goodyear-Bruch, RN, PhD, CCRN

DECEMBER 30

"Intensive care units and other specialized units score higher in nurse-physician relationships than do less specialized units."

–Claudia Schmalenberg, RN, MSN, and Marlene Kramer, RN, PhD
From "Nurse-Physician Relationships in Hospitals:
20,000 Nurses Tell Their Story" (Critical Care Nurse, *Vol.29/*
No.1; pp 74-83)

DECEMBER 31

CLINICAL PEARL

Always consider increased intracranial pressure when there
is a change in a patient's level of consciousness.

Patricia Vanderpool, MSN, APN-BC, ANPE

Bibliography

American Association of Critical Care Nurses (n.d.). *The 4 A's to rise above moral distress.* Retrieved November 15, 2009 from http://www.aacn.org/WD/Practice/Docs/4As_to_Rise_Above_Moral_Distress.pdf

American Association of Critical Care Nurses (2005). AACN standards for establishing and sustaining healthy work environments: A journey to excellence. *American Journal of Critical Care, 14,* 187-197.

Boyd, N. (2004). May. In S. Hudacek (Ed.), *A daybook for nurses: Making a difference each day* (p. 62). Indianapolis, IN: Sigma Theta Tau International.

Briskin, A., & Boller, J. (2006). *Daily miracles: Stories and practices of humanity and excellence in health care.* Indianapolis, IN: Sigma Theta Tau International.

Dickenson-Hazard, N. (2008). *Ready, set, go lead! A primer for emerging health care leaders.* Indianapolis, IN: Sigma Theta Tau International.

Doherty, K. (2004). April. In S. Hudacek (Ed.), *A daybook for nurses: Making a difference each day* (p. 84). Indianapolis, IN: Sigma Theta Tau International.

Elders, J. (2006). July. In Sigma Theta Tau International, *A daybook for nurse leaders and mentors* (p. 84). Indianapolis, IN: Author.

Godshall, M. (2004). February. In S. Hudacek (Ed.), *A daybook for nurses: Making a difference each day.* Indianapolis, IN: Sigma Theta Tau International.

Haidt, J. (2005). *The happiness hypothesis: Finding modern truth in ancient wisdom.* New York: Basic Books

Hillesum, E. (2009). Stress. In S. Weinstein, *B is for balance* (p. 37). Indianapolis, IN: Sigma Theta Tau International.

Hudacek, S. (2004). *A daybook for nurses: Making a difference each day.* Indianapolis, IN: Sigma Theta Tau International.

Hudacek, S. (2004). *Making a difference: Stories from the point of care: Vo. 2.* Indianapolis, IN: Sigma Theta Tau International.

Hudacek, S. (2005). *Making a difference: Stories from the point of care: Vol. 1.* Indianapolis, IN: Sigma Theta Tau International.

Kasiak-Gambla, J. (2004). October. In S. Hudacek (Ed.), *A daybook for nurses: Making a difference each day* (p. 120). Indianapolis, IN: Sigma Theta Tau International.

Kirchhoff, K., Palzkill, J., Kowalkowski, J., Mork, A., & Gretarsdottir, E. (2008). Preparing families of intensive care patients for withdrawal of life support: A pilot study. *American Journal of Critical Care, 17*(2), 113-121.

Lopes, C. (2004). June. In S. Hudacek (Ed.), *A daybook for nurses: Making a difference each day* (p. 70). Indianapolis, IN: Sigma Theta Tau International.

McAdam, J. L., & Puntillo, K. (2009). Symptoms experienced by family members of patients in intensive care units. *American Journal of Critical Care, 18*(3), 200-210.

Munro, C. (2009). Hope and change in critical care. *American Journal of Critical Care, 18,* 188-190.

NeSmith, E. G., Weinrich, S. P., Andrews, J. O., Medeiros, R. S., Hawkins, M. L., & Weinrich, M. (2009). Systemic inflammatory response syndrome score and race as predictors of length of stay in the intensive care unit. *American Journal of Critical Care, 18*(4), 339-347.

O'Meara, D., Mireles-Cabodevila, E., Frame, F., Hummell, A. C., Hammel, J., & Dweik, R. A., et al. (2008). Evaluation of delivery of enteral nutrition in critically ill patients receiving mechanical ventilation. *American Journal of Critical Care, 17*(1), 53-61.

Perme, C., & Chandrashekar, R. (2009). Early mobility and walking program for patients in intensive care units: Creating a standard of care. *American Journal of Critical Care, 18*(3), 212-221.

Pesut, D. (2006). August. In Sigma Theta Tau International, *A daybook for nurse leaders and mentors* (p. 103). Indianapolis, IN: Author.

Prendergast, V., Hallberg, I. R., Jahnke, H ., Kleiman, C., & Hagell, P. (2009). Oral health, ventilator-associated pneumonia, and intracranial pressure in intubated patients in a neuroscience intensive care unit. *American Journal of Critical Care, 18*(4), 368-376.

Riches, A. (2004). April. In S. Hudacek (Ed.), *A daybook for nurses: Making a difference each day* (p. 54). Indianapolis, IN: Sigma Theta Tau International.

Santley, E. (2004). April. In S. Hudacek (Ed.), *A daybook for nurses: Making a difference each day* (p. 46). Indianapolis, IN: Sigma Theta Tau International.

Schaffer, M., & Norlander, L. (2009). *Being present: A nurse's resource for end-of-life communication.* Indianapolis, IN: Sigma Theta Tau International.

Schmalenberg, C., & Kramer, M. (2009). Nurse-physician relationships in hospitals: 20,000 nurses tell their story. *Critical Care Nurse, 29*(1), 74-83.

Sherman, S. (2007). Mentors and mentees: An interview with Susan Sherman. In In T. Hansen-Turton, S. Sherman, & V. Ferguson (Eds.), *Conversations with leaders: Frank talk from nurses (and others) on the front lines of leadership* (pp. 144-16). Indianapolis, IN: Sigma Theta Tau International.

Sigma Theta Tau International (2006). *Daybook for nurse leaders and mentors.* Indianapolis, IN: Author.

Sole, M. L., Aragon Penoyer, D., Su, X., Jimenez, E., Kalita, S. J., Poalillo, E., et al. (2209). Assessment of endotracheal cuff pressure by continuous monitoring: A pilot study. *American Journal of Critical Care, 18*(2), 133-143.

Twibell, R. S., Siela, D., Riwitis, C., Wheatley, J., Riegle, T., & Bousman, D., et al. (2008). Nurses perception about the benefits of family presence during resuscitation. *American Journal of Critical Care, 17*(2), 101-111.

Watson, J. (2007). Conversations and reflections on my journey into the heart of nursing: Human caring-healing. In T. Hansen-Turton, S. Sherman, & V. Ferguson (Eds.), *Conversations with leaders: Frank talk from nurses (and others) on the front lines of leadership* (pp. 174-183). Indianapolis, IN: Sigma Theta Tau International.

Weinstein, S. (2009). *B is for balance.* Indianapolis, IN: Sigma Theta Tau International.

Yee, C. (2004). March. In S. Hudacek (Ed.), *A daybook for nurses: Making a difference each day* (p. 33). Indianapolis, IN: Sigma Theta Tau International.

Index of Authors

*Names marked with an asterisk (*) indicate past presidents of the American Association of Critical-Care Nurses who graciously contributed their writings for this project.

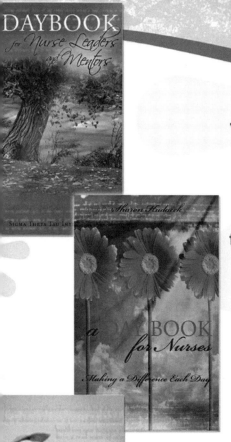
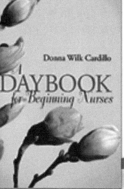

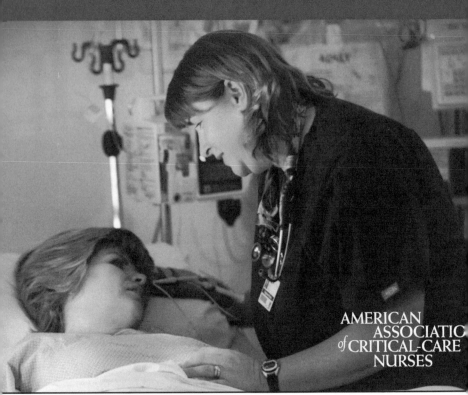
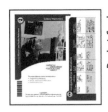
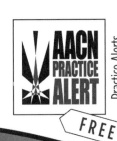
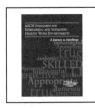